IT'S MORE THAN JUST A HEADACHE . . .

* I can't stand any kind of bright light during an attack.
* I notice that certain smells make my migraine worse.
* All I want to do is lie down in a dark room.
* During my attack even my skin hurts. Is that my imagination?
* Why do I feel so nauseated when I get a headache?
* I feel like I'm going crazy with these visions. Is there a physical reason behind them?
* I just want to die during attacks.

**AND THERES MORE THAN JUST AN
ASPIRIN FOR RELIEF . . .
FIND OUT WHAT YOU CAN DO IN—**

MIGRAINES
Everything You Need to Know About Their Cause and Cure

MIGRAINES

EVERYTHING YOU NEED TO KNOW ABOUT THEIR CAUSE AND CURE

ARTHUR ELKIND, M.D.

AVON BOOKS ◆ NEW YORK

The ideas, procedures, and suggestions in this book are intended to supplement, not replace, the medical advice of a trained medical professional. All matters regarding your health require medical supervision. Consult your physician before adopting the suggestions in this book, as well as any condition that may require diagnosis or medical attention. The author and publisher disclaim any liability arising directly or indirectly from the use of this book.

AVON BOOKS
A division of
The Hearst Corporation
1350 Avenue of the Americas
New York, New York 10019

Copyright © 1997 by CMD Publishing, a division of Current Medical Directions, Inc.
Published by arrangement with CMD Publishing, a division of Current Medical Directions, Inc.
Visit our website at **http://AvonBooks.com**
Library of Congress Catalog Card Number 97-93166
ISBN: 0-380-79077-7

First Avon Books Printing: October 1997

Printed in the U.S.A.

WCD 10 9 8 7 6 5 4

Contents

Chapter 1
What Is Migraine?   1

Chapter 2
The Migraine Attack   17

Chapter 3
The Causes of Migraine: A Biological Short-Circuit   36

Chapter 4
The Common Triggers of Migraine   56

Chapter 5
Migraine and Women: The Estrogen Connection   78

Chapter 6
The Young Migraine Sufferer   92

Chapter 7
The Treatment Approach   111

Chapter 8
Drug Therapy   131

Chapter 9
Alternatives to Drug Treatment for Migraine   155

Chapter 10
Living with Migraine   178

Charts:
Modified Headache Classification Chart   194
Headache Disability Rating   196
Common Headache Triggers   197

Glossary   205

Bibliography   217

Beyond This Book: Resources for
Headache Sufferers   232

Index   241

ONE

What Is Migraine?

CASE STUDY

When Barbara and her daughter Ann arrived at my clinic, I could see the family resemblance in their worried expressions. Barbara had experienced her first migraine over twenty-five years ago and had been suffering silently all that time. The family knew that she often got headaches and sometimes had to retreat to a dark, quiet room, but they had no idea just how awful the attacks were. She had never consulted with a headache specialist or neurologist. During regular checkups, she only occasionally mentioned her "sick headaches," and quietly accepted advice from doctors along the lines of "lie down until it's over." Even when she started getting aura—the group of visual or other perceptual disturbances associated with migraine—ranging from black spots to florid visions, the prescription didn't change. As Barbara recalls, "I couldn't believe it. I had just seen a giraffe walk through the living room and my doctor simply told me to take two aspirin!" Still, she trusted the family physician, who claimed the pain and visions were a hysterical reaction to stress, and resigned herself to the agony.

But the day her 21-year-old daughter came home crying from work, complaining of terrible pain and constant nausea, Barbara's attitude toward migraine changed. "It was okay for me to suffer," she said, "but there's no way my little girl was going to go through what I did!" Barbara went to her primary care physician and for the first time demanded

1

to know, "What is this awful problem, and what can we do about it?" She was referred to me.

That first day, Barbara, Ann, and I talked about migraine—what it was and how it might be treated. Then we went to work. Barbara's migraine attacks proved easy to treat. They were clearly linked to certain food triggers. She kept a headache diary that helped define a trigger-free diet. By the end of the year, Barbara's biweekly headaches had been reduced to one every month or so, and medication effectively stopped the pain of those. Ann is still working on her treatment, since her triggers proved harder to identify, but now she knows there's hope. Today, both mother and daughter feel in control of their migraine.

"Exactly what *is* a migraine—and do I have it?"

By the time you reach a headache clinic, you may have asked that question any number of times and received any number of answers. No one can see a headache, so its diagnosis and treatment are highly subjective—the result of trial and error, judicious examination, and a careful review of a person's headache history. I've been treating migraine for thirty years now. I've seen headaches of every type and every conceivable symptom. Yet migraine can still fascinate and amaze physicians who treat it daily. Each migraine sufferer is highly individual. His or her symptoms and the way he or she manages this complex disorder are often unique.

But while a doctor may see migraine as an intriguing challenge, the people who suffer from this condition find it excruciatingly painful, debilitating, even embarrassing at times. It's common to be greeted with raised eyebrows from doctors as well as laymen when complaining about the severity of the disorder. Most people simply do not understand how serious and debilitating it is. Economic loss to individuals and business measures in the billions.

Aside from migraine's effects on a sufferer's work life, it can cause other disruptions in lifestyle as well. The disorder can be quirky, taking forms other than a painful headache. Patients often feel nauseated or vomit; they may experience light sensitivity or have other vision impairments, numbness, and even temporary paralysis. They may see things, even smell things, that simply aren't there.

All of which helps to explain the fact that many people approach the subject of their own migraine with guilt, shame, and fear. They face the constant skepticism of family, friends, and co-workers over their "invisible" symptoms. They meet the headache specialist while harboring secret fears of brain tumors or psychosis: "Will the doctor discover I'm fatally ill? Will my physician think I'm crazy?" And through it all, they look at their own symptoms and wonder, "All this from a *migraine*?"

The answer is yes. Migraine is a diffuse kind of disorder that affects many organs and manifests itself in many different ways. Most people have common headache, but there are many who fall outside of the ordinary, which has made the classification of migraine difficult for many years.

In fact, it was only in recent decades that doctors finally agreed on the classifications of migraine. For centuries, headache had been something of a hodgepodge of diagnoses without any real organization. Its criteria could vary from one physician to the next. Then, in 1962, a group of headache specialists met to determine some standard classifications. They decided on the terms "common," for the frequently encountered migraine without aura, and "classic," for the less common migraine with aura. Other types of headache were classified as well.

Those classifications remained the standard until the International Headache Society redefined headache disorders in 1988. That international committee of neurologists and headache specialists recategorized migraine in light of new discoveries and treatments. The terms classic and common were officially dropped, although they still show up today in discussions on migraine. What remained were "migraine with aura" and "migraine without aura." Other headache types were redefined in the classifications at that time also, including cluster headache and tension-type headache. Although these classifications may change as we learn more about migraine, the 1988 standards are used by specialists today, and will likely shape a doctor's diagnosis of your own migraine.

Yet, even with clear classifications, specialists still see many migraineurs—or migraine sufferers—who come in and say, "My doctor says it can't be migraine." I recall one woman in particular who always had a headache on the same side of her head. Her doctor examined her for sinus and dental disease. But when she came to me, I realized that she had all the symptoms of migraine, including nausea and light sensitivity. The only thing out of the ordinary was that the headaches always occurred on the same side of her head. In some cases, migraine attacks may mask other illnesses. You have to be sure you're not dealing with something else, especially when the symptoms fall outside the ordinary. After performing tests to rule out all the things that can mimic the disorder, I knew that this particular woman did indeed have migraine. She responded beautifully to treatment and has very few migraine headaches now.

There is no need to suffer silently from migraine, no more than you would from severe respiratory infection or other diseases. Gathering information on migraine should be your first step in the battle for control over the disorder. Your first line of defense: Learn what migraine is and how to recognize it.

What is a migraine? Is there a simple definition?

Mi-graine: a condition that is marked by recurrent, usually unilateral severe headache often accompanied by nausea and vomiting and followed by sleep, that tends to occur in more than one member of a family, and that is of uncertain origin though attacks appear to be precipitated by dilation of intracranial blood vessels.

—*Webster's Third New International Dictionary*

Medically speaking, migraine is what's termed a benign, recurrent disorder. Simply speaking, that means migraine is a treatable ailment that, while often extremely painful, is not essentially dangerous. Like every medical ailment, migraine has its signature symptoms. By far the most prevalent of these is a moderate to severe headache, a pulsating pain that may persist anywhere from four hours to as many as three days. As a rule, migraine headaches are unilateral, or one-sided, affecting only half the head during an attack, although the side that feels pain may vary. But migraine is more than just a headache. Nausea, vomiting, light sensitivity, and sound sensitivity are all symptoms, and there are others that are less common. Finally, in roughly 15 to 20 percent of diagnosed cases, migraine attacks are associated with aura that occurs in the moments before headache pain begins.

What is an aura?

Aura is the term used to describe a large group of visual or other perceptual disturbances associated with migraine. About one migraine attack in five exhibits this symptom. Aura most often makes an appearance in the moments before an attack, but occasionally pops up during headache. Aura can be one of migraine's most intriguing—and alarming—symptoms. Often a person suffers quietly with migraine headaches for years, never seeing a doctor, but the initial appearance of an aura sends him or her speeding to a specialist for the first time. The most classic form of aura is a vision of zigzagging lines around a darkened center. These lines are called *fortification spectra*, in reference to the medieval fort structures they resemble, and are a type of aura known as *teichopsia*. Other aura reported are shooting stars of light, called *photopsia*. Some migraine sufferers experience distorted perceptions of their bodies. These distortions, which can make people feel very small (*micropsia*), or very large (*macropsia*), are not uncommon in young people. Other migraineurs lose a quarter or even half of their normal field of vision. Images outside of that field of vision seem to disappear in what's termed *negative scotoma*. Some auras border on delusions or hallucinations: they appear as sounds or smells that aren't really there. Some people smell perfume or some other pleasant—or unpleasant—odor. Others describe a numbness that makes them feel like a dentist has injected half their mouth with painkillers. Lips might be numb prior to a headache; that's very characteristic of an aura. Often, people have numbness in their hand or fingers on the same side as the numbness in their face. Some even describe a weakness, however transient, akin to paralysis. Some people black out. These physical disturbances are called *sensory aura*. Aura can be quite variable, manifesting itself not just through vision but through other areas of perception as well. (For more about aura, see Chapter 2, ''The Migraine Attack.'')

What if my attacks don't match that simple definition? Does that mean I don't have migraines?

Migraine is quite complex, and its symptoms may vary considerably from one person to another. A general definition of migraine doesn't allow for the highly unique way it can manifest itself in certain sufferers. Your headaches may last for many hours or may vanish after a few brief but incredibly painful minutes, and still be symptoms of migraine. They may disappear for months or show up with such regularity that you can set your clock by them. Headache pain tends to be one-sided, but occasionally a migraineur may experience it on both sides of the head. Migraine headaches may strike at any time of the day or night; they might even wake you from a sound sleep. Some migraine attacks begin with headaches so agonizing that they make sufferers suicidal; other people report no head pain at all, but are still correctly identified as having migraine (see migraine variants on page 12). Just because the disorder takes many forms does not mean it can't be diagnosed and controlled.

How do I know if I have migraine or just ordinary headaches?

Migraine is a disorder; headache is simply a symptom of that disorder. It's the most common symptom, so it is most often associated with migraine and is sometimes confused for the disorder itself. However, think of migraine as being a condition like diabetes. Sugar in the urine is a sign of diabetes; diabetes is the primary disorder associated with it. But it's only one sign. There are also kidney, heart, eye, and neurological disturbances that go along with diabetes. These are the condition's other symptoms—just as headache is only one part of migraine. Migraine is a multiple syndrome that involves a wide variety of symptoms. There may be nausea, vomiting, or effects on the nervous system, stomach, heart, and eyes. Therefore, in order for a doctor to make a diagnosis of migraine, typically you would have to have at least one of the following symptoms in addition to head pain: sensitivity to light, sensitivity to sound, nausea, or vomiting. It's important to remember, though, that this is not a diagnosis that you can make on your own—only a doctor can do that.

What are the different types of headache?

There are many different types of headache outlined in the classification chart adopted by the International Headache Society in 1988. More have been defined by individual physicians in subsequent modified charts. But in most discussions, headache tends to get lumped into a few broad categories: migraine, with its two subclassifications of migraine with aura and migraine without aura; cluster headache; tension-type headache; complicated migraine; and, finally, the least common forms of migraine, which could include disorders like the relatively rare familial hemiplegic migraine.

Is there a foolproof test for migraine?

No. So far, tests are no substitute for a careful examination and a review of your personal headache history by a qualified physician. Testing doesn't pinpoint migraine—it rules out other diseases and helps your doctor narrow down the field of options. By learning your family medical history and analyzing your personal account of past attacks, a doctor can produce a diagnosis that is far more reliable than any test. However, expect to undergo some screening when you go for treatment, if only to eliminate other possible biological factors. Tests may include CAT (computerized axial tomography) scans, neuroimaging, laboratory tests, or psychological evaluations. You'll read more about these examinations in Chapter 7, "The Treatment Approach."

Who gets migraine?

The statistics vary. That may be due to the fact that until quite recently, doctors didn't agree on what could be classified as migraine, so historical data is not reliable. However, the *Journal of the American Medical Association* (*JAMA*) recently published a study based on a new survey that indicates that twenty-three million Americans have migraine—that's 8 percent of the total population. That's enough people to populate the states of Alaska, Arizona, Maine, Maryland, North Carolina, South Carolina, and Oregon. Other estimates place the number as high as fifty million. The study in *JAMA* confirmed that migraine is most common between the ages of twenty to fifty, while numbers decline significantly in older age groups. However, you can still find sufferers among people over the age of fifty, and in children as well. Most migraineurs report having at least one relative who also experiences attacks. That relative is usually the person's mother.

When does migraine first strike?

Most people get their first attack before the age of forty, with one-third of all sufferers reporting onset of migraine by the age of ten. Toddlers as young as a year-and-a-half have been diagnosed with headache, and younger children may also get them but be unable to successfully articulate their pain. Other sufferers may not experience an attack until they reach their seventies or eighties. Circumstances like those are not all that common, however.

Is it true that people with lower incomes get fewer migraines?

That's one of the long-held theories on migraine shattered by the results of *JAMA*'s recent study. It seems that people with lower incomes are actually *more* likely to suffer from migraine attacks. Stress is a common trigger of migraine, so it shouldn't be surprising that people who are struggling financially suffer from migraine more often. In addition, the life and diet changes needed to eliminate other potential triggers may not be an option for people with limited financial resources. Finally, medical treatment may not be as accessible.

Is it true that migraine attacks are a sign of intelligence and only affect smart or creative people?

Migraine can strike anyone, of any level of intellect. But you may draw comfort from the fact that through the years many highly creative and influential people have suffered from migraine. As a migraineur, you share company with political and military leaders like Julius Caesar, Peter the Great, Queen Mary Tudor, General Ulysses S. Grant, Thomas Jefferson, and Woodrow Wilson. Creative geniuses like Lewis Carroll, Frederic Chopin, Virginia Woolf, Edgar Allan Poe, Peter Tchaikovsky, Sigmund Freud, Blaise Pascal, Elizabeth Barrett Browning, and George Bernard Shaw all had migraine. For these authors and artists, migraine may have played a part in shaping their unique visions. Mystics, seers, and figures from the Bible like Saint Paul can credit aura for enhancing some of their visions. Scientists like Alexander Graham Bell, Alfred Nobel, and Charles Darwin had migraine. Basketball great Kareem Abdul-Jabbar is another migraineur.

Is migraine strictly an American phenomenon?

Not at all. Virtually every industrialized nation has similar migraine statistics. Less industrialized countries report fewer numbers of migraineurs, but these statistics can be deceiving. They may simply reflect a lack of adequate medical care and a subsequent drop in the number of people correctly diagnosed with this disorder, or a different set of standards may be applied when classifying migraine. People may also be hesitant to report migraine in societies where such conditions might be misunderstood, or even ridiculed, rather than treated.

When is a migraine dangerous? Are the headaches damaging my brain?

Unless caused by a neurological disease, which is relatively rare, migraine is not dangerous. It may feel like your head is being squeezed in a vise, but there is no evidence to support the idea that migraine has any permanent effect on your brain.

Should I just suffer quietly? Or do I need to see a doctor?

Don't just "take it." Instead, take control of your migraine. By monitoring your food intake and eliminating migraine triggers that a doctor helps you to identify, you may reduce the severity or frequency of your attacks by half. Anyone suffering from migraine should see a doctor about his or her head pain at least once in his or her lifetime, if only to eliminate other biological factors like hypertension, an aneurysm, or a brain tumor. Although the odds of your migraine being caused by one of those diseases may be slim, it's not a risk you should take. Get a diagnosis from a doctor. Learning that your pain has a benign biological origin may relieve some of your feelings of stress—one of migraine's most common triggers. The visit alone can be a significant step toward managing your migraine.

What is complicated migraine?

With complicated migraine, a person has neurological symptoms that occur before or during the headache and last well after the headache itself has disappeared. These symptoms might include speech difficulty, visual difficulty, paralysis, milder forms of paralysis, or sensory disturbances. A person may have numbness or tingling in the face and limbs that can continue for a prolonged period of time.

How important is it to know what kind of migraine I have? Will knowing that help?

There's no question that identifying your migraine type will help, but only because classifying a headache is an integral part of treating it. Once you know what kind of migraine you have, you and your doctor can target your efforts to combat it. For example, there's clear evidence to show that some drugs work better fighting cluster headache than others. Clearly those would be the first line of defense if your headache is classified as such. Rebound headache—which is thought to occur when a headache sufferer overuses his or her medication—would merit a look at the type and amounts of medication taken. If your headaches are found to be associated with head trauma, then the trauma should be addressed, and your headaches will be affected by the treatment you receive. Classifying your headache and giving it a name will help both you and your doctor manage your health care more efficiently.

My daughter suffers from basilar migraine. What kind of migraine is that?

Basilar artery migraine involves branches of the basilar artery. A spasm of these arteries can cause decreased blood flow to the back of the brain. The result is weakness in the lower extremities, nausea and vomiting, dizziness, blurred vision, and blackouts. It often occurs in young menstruating women, sometimes starting in adolescence. Some of these sufferers become so ill that their physicians refer them for a neurological workup, thinking it may be a brain tumor or other disease. This idea is dispelled when the pain goes away and comes back repeatedly. A close look at a person's medical history may indicate a benign, though often debilitating, basilar artery migraine.

Cluster headaches sound ominous. What are they?

Unfortunately, cluster headache is every bit as unpleasant as it sounds. As its name suggests, it attacks in groups or waves. Cluster headaches are related to migraine, although doctors still aren't clear on the connection. What makes cluster headache fascinating is that it's very often an instantaneous diagnosis. When the person comes in, it's nearly always a male with an excruciatingly severe, one-sided headache. The story is usually the same: Horrible pains wake him up between two and four o'clock in the morning. The pain can affect the face, involving one eye and radiating back toward the ear, in what is known as the temporal region. That region covers what is essentially a quarter of the head: Draw an imaginary line down the middle of the nose, right below the eye, then drag it back at least as far as the ear. People who suffer from cluster headache feel excruciating, stabbing pain in that whole area. The attack lasts approximately forty-five minutes. Finally, the person can go back to sleep, only to awaken again with another attack. It's called cluster because the attacks arrive in waves, lasting for about four to six weeks, once or twice a year. The headaches occur two to ten times a day. Obviously this can be very disturbing. During the period of cluster, attacks follow a bell-shaped curve. In other words, they begin slowly, with a gradual increase in pain, and then, toward the end of the cycle, the pain tapers off. For an interim of six to eight months, the person feels fine. This cycle is repeated endlessly if the cluster headache is not treated. With a doctor's assistance, the cycle can be cut off or its bell shape changed for the better.

What treatments exist for cluster headaches?

There are drugs used to combat cluster headaches before they establish their cycle. They include ergots and medications with lithium; Catapres, DHE-45, Depakote, and Xylocaine are other medications used in the treatment of cluster.

Imitrex is also a potential drug treatment for these cyclical headaches. Nondrug treatments include inhaling pure oxygen—this is tremendously effective. New research is being done on the use of bright-light therapy; ask your doctor about the latest information on this treatment. As a last resort, there is a surgery called radio-frequency trigeminal gangliolysis; however, side effects of this procedure, such as loss of some sensory perception, are permanent and often unpleasant.

How can I tell if I have a tension-type headache?

Tension-type headache is the most common of all headaches. It is what may be termed a regular or everyday headache, which occurs with stress or other factors. Perhaps 75 to 80 percent of the population suffers from tension-type headache at one time or another. Tension-type headache lacks most of the symptoms associated with migraine, such as nausea or light sensitivity. No one is quite sure what mechanism brings on tension-type headache. Put simply, we know that tension can be manifested in muscle contractions that affect blood vessels and bring on head pain. When stressed, you might actually feel your neck muscles tighten up, along with the muscles in your shoulders and scalp. Then it feels as if you're wearing a hat that's too tight, or that someone is tightening a band around your head with malignant twists of a screw. However, it's mostly a superficial kind of headache. Unlike migraine, it isn't due to a change that takes place in the brain or the surface of the brain; it's centered in the scalp and the muscles on the outside of the skull. Many people get tension-type headache in addition to migraine. A tension-type headache sometimes precedes a migraine attack. Generally, tension-type headache can be self-treated by taking over-the-counter drugs like ibuprofen, aspirin, or acetaminophen. A cup of coffee and an aspirin are a combination that has been known to work.

What is a migraine variant?

Variant types of headaches are linked to symptoms that are associated with the urinary tract (i.e., kidneys, bladder) rather than the more classic migraine symptoms of head pain and, perhaps, aura. It's thought that in some cases, variants such as nausea or vomiting may replace head pain. This is particularly true in young people. Children often suffer from abdominal pain, nausea, and vomiting. In situations where the doctor can't find anything organically wrong, and the children also have histories of headaches at other times, it's thought they might have a migraine variant.

How do you measure the severity of a headache?

The severity of migraine is usually rated by its impact on your normal range of activities. Your migraine can be judged by these criteria:

- *Mild*: Attacks do not interfere with your daily routine.
- *Moderate*: Attacks limit activities, but less than half of your routine is affected.
- *Moderately severe*: Your activities are limited by more than 50 percent during an attack, and migraine is highly disruptive of your life.
- *Severe*: You are so debilitated by the attacks, you are forced to lie down for two or more hours during an episode, and your activities remain limited for hours or even days after an attack.

Most migraine attacks are moderate to severe. Tension-type headaches more often fall into the mild to moderate range. Cluster headaches, on the other hand, are usually severe.

Can you get a migraine every day?

If someone gets a headache every day, it's not usually a migraine. It's called a chronic daily headache, and can usually be traced to muscle tension, anxiety, and sometimes rebound headache. Most people have only occasional headache. I've treated people who get only one migraine attack a year. It arrives with classic aura—visual symptoms and zigzag lines—it lasts a while, then goes away. It doesn't come back for another twelve months. Other people get headache once or twice a week. The average number of attacks for people with migraine is one to three headaches a month, most often on weekends.

What is a rebound headache?

Some people use headache medication too frequently, and it's thought that these drugs cause headaches to come back—or rebound—when the medication has been absorbed into the body. In other words, it had been shown that certain medications, both over-the-counter and prescription, when overused for headache, can create a desire on the part of the brain, a craving for more of the medicine. This is called a reward system. The system starts off with the drug initially giving relief—the reward. Then, as use of the drug increases, the brain needs the reward more often. Unfortunately, in order to satisfy itself, the brain gives the signal of headache and pain—creating rebound—so it can get more of the drug. Oddly enough, many people who take these same compounds for joint pains or arthritis don't get rebound pain, so the reward system isn't the sole answer to the question of what causes rebound.

Why do my headaches seem to come in regular cycles?

No one knows why some headaches are more regular than others, although a recognized link between menstrual cycles and migraine in many female headache patients may be one explanation. (See Chapter 5, ''Migraine and Women: The Estrogen Connection.'') Other people's migraine cycles may be defined by time of day, month, or year. Still others report attacks that are random.

My migraines last for days and days. How common is that?

On average, most migraine attacks last from four hours to as long as three days, so you're not alone. Often, a person experiences weakness and lethargy, a ''headache hangover,'' which can last for a day or two after the migraine attack. With complicated migraine, the symptoms felt during headache—including nausea, vomiting, light sensitivity, and numbness or cold sensations in the feet and hands—can persist even after all pain has gone.

Does headache occurrence have any link with race, like some other diseases?

There is some evidence to show that African-Americans get migraine less often than Caucasians. Studies on this are still open for interpretation. One theory is that African-Americans have higher levels of a certain enzyme in their blood. This enzyme targets tyramine, an amino acid that may play a role in the opening and closing of blood vessels in the brain. Tyramine crops up in foods that can trigger headache, such as aged cheese and wine.

Are more people getting migraine than ever before?

We know that people have been getting migraine since the first century B.C., and undoubtedly for centuries prior to that. Archeological evidence suggests that radical treatment for migraine—drilling holes into people's skulls—was being performed as far back as 2,500 years ago. In the thirteenth century, describing your aura to a friend might have landed you on a burning stake as a witch. With "treatment" options like that, many people probably chose to remain silent about their disorder. Documentation even as late as this century is also sketchy, because studies weren't conducted specifically on migraine occurrence. It cropped up as a secondary disorder in other surveys, but good research studies and surveys that specifically target migraine sufferers have not been done until recently. It may seem like more people are getting them now simply because people are more open about discussing this health issue than ever before.

Will this whole thing just go away?

Headache pain tends to fade as people get older. After the age of fifty or sixty, migraine occurrence usually decreases, if it doesn't go away completely. In the meantime, your migraine is probably not going anywhere without some help from a doctor and some concentrated effort from you. While attacks can be controlled or alleviated with drugs, it's crucial to avoid your particular migraine triggers—the foods or situations that seem to bring on your attacks—and reduce the stress in your life.

As a male who suffers from migraines, I feel like an endangered species. People are skeptical. What can I do to get them to take my pain seriously?

People are probably reacting to the fact that more women than men suffer from migraine, at a ratio of three to one.

However, that's no reason for anyone to doubt your claims of pain. Men in particular are likely candidates for cluster headache. You might share the statistics on job loss and economic costs with these skeptics: The total bill for lost work time, health care, and medication for headache disorders in America alone amounts to roughly six to eight billion a year. Over half of the twenty-three million American migraine sufferers estimated by the *JAMA* study have headaches so severe that they can't work or conduct their normal activities while an attack is in progress. If that doesn't convince others of the seriousness of your condition, remember that people are more likely to take your pain seriously if you do. If people observe that you conscientiously avoid headache triggers, that you consult a doctor or specialist, and stay up-to-date on treatments and drug information, they may respond more sympathetically to your claims.

Some people say, "It's only a headache, just deal with it." I get so angry I don't even know what to say to them. How can I respond to people like that?

Ask them how they "deal" with the pain of a bad back or a painful tooth. Then ask them how they would handle that pain if it persisted for hours or days at a time—and no drug or treatment could make it go away. If it's a friend or family member, invite them to stick around during an attack. Let them see the physical toll that migraine takes on its sufferers. Migraine is a vascular (blood vessel) disorder with *physical* effects. Fortunately, there are people on your side who won't say, "It's only a headache." You can find doctors and other sufferers who take your pain as seriously as you do. Seek them out. Share your story with people who understand, and it will be easier to shrug off those who deny your pain. An additional benefit of making contact with headache support networks and doctors is that you may be able to obtain literature that points out the very debilitating nature of the disorder, including statistics that show it's a significant cause of lost work and leisure time. Share the literature with co-workers and friends.

❧

TWO

The Migraine Attack

CASE STUDY

Jo had grown used to tension-type headaches by the time she got to college. Every few weeks she'd get that dull pain spreading up from her neck. It usually went away with a few aspirin. Jo began taking birth control pills, and one day she doubled over in class, barely making it to her room before vomiting. "I just huddled under a blanket in my room, crying, crying, for almost two days," she remembers. "It was like no other headache I'd had before." Her doctor took her off the pills, but neither he nor Jo ever considered migraine—they both attributed the pain to a side effect of the pills.

Then it struck repeatedly. This went on for a few years. Each time, Jo blamed the flu or food poisoning, until she had an attack every week for a month—each attack of pain felt as if a knife was rhythmically stabbing deep into her brain. Terrified that something was deadly wrong, Jo was too afraid to have her worst fears confirmed by a doctor. But one Friday night the pain was so bad, Jo was sure that an aneurysm had just exploded in her head. In tears, she tried to drive to the emergency room but could hardly stagger to the car. A neighbor took her to the hospital. Jo's speech was slurred, and pain radiated through her if she so much as moved her head to one side. In a daze she answered questions and watched emergency room personnel inject her with a migraine medication. Jo was stunned that they thought it was migraine. She was even more shocked when the pain went away.

That Monday, Jo made a beeline for the clinic. Jo told me that right before the latest attack, her vision had dissolved into pieces, like looking through a kaleidoscope. Her hands went cold and her mind went blank. "I couldn't even read the numbers on the phone," Jo said. "Nothing seemed to make sense." The rest of Jo's history of attacks confirmed what the emergency personnel had suspected: Jo had a classic case of migraine.

Whenever two or more migraine sufferers meet, it's the same—the immediate swap of symptoms and descriptions of their attacks, followed by surprise over the wildly varied forms that migraine takes. These meetings can sometimes raise more questions than they answer: Are my symptoms normal, or are theirs?

Just as your fingerprints are unique, so, too, are migraine attacks. Yet, there are many traits and phases that crop up over and over in migraineurs' accounts.

Some of the best descriptions of migraine attacks and their classic symptoms come from a woman who didn't even recognize her attacks for what they were. A Benedictine abbess living in the 1100s, named Hildegard of Bingen, wrote extensively of her chronic illnesses, religious visions, and horrifying dreams, little realizing that centuries later doctors would make a diagnosis: They were all the result of migraine. Hildegard viewed some of these experiences, such as the aura visions, as a gift from God. She made spiritual interpretations of the images she saw: Flashing lights became the "Living Flame" of God, zigzag lines formed a building that could be both protective and imprisoning. The blindness interrupting a field of view during an attack was interpreted by Hildegard as the abyss and darkness of ignorance and sin. Hildegard regarded other symptoms with the same horror and despair common to migraine patients today, only she perceived them as the work of a dark authority rather than as a biological disorder linked to overworked blood vessels.

Hildegard's unique ability to shape her symptoms to a higher purpose is not easily shared by most sufferers, but we can still learn a lot about headache management from this twelfth-century mystic. She turned the symptoms to good use where she could, worked with herbs and other medicines to reduce the pain, went to bed when the pain became unbearable, and went on with her life in the periods between bouts—cramming as much living as she could into those days and months.

Perhaps you share the two types of visions the abbess described—the dark dreams of the preattack, or prodrome, phase, and the more colorful, florid images of aura. The aura inspired Hildegard. She used her knowledge of religious texts to interpret the aura's glowing images. But the prodrome dreams disturbed her, causing her to ask the same anxious questions most migraineurs do, although in slightly more flowery style.

> . . . These dreams that are plaguing me come only when I am deeply, nearly deathly asleep, in a sleep that is both deeper and more troubled than is normal for me. . . . These dreams are different: unclear and confusing, without any interpreting voice, they are never direct with me. What is their relationship to me? Is it possible they could be of the devil? Of course, this is what I fear most and what has prevented me from speaking of them as yet.

Patients are afraid to name many symptoms they experience during an attack, even to their closest family and friends. Don't be afraid to share your symptoms with others or admit them to yourself. They may seem bizarre, but chances are, they're common. Do you see things or smell things that aren't there? Are you strangely tired or alarmingly energized for days around an attack? Are your hands numb? Does pain arrive at 8 a.m., every single morning, like clockwork? Does your vision fragment, swirl, and dissolve into surrealistic images? Ask yourself these questions, and in this chapter you'll find the answer to the one that usually follows: Is this *normal*?

What is a typical migraine attack like?

In a "typical" migraine attack there are essentially four stages: the preattack phase, known as prodrome; the aura stage, with its visions and other sensory disturbances; then the headache pain itself; and finally the postdrome, or postheadache, phase. After these four phases, your migraine attack is over and you feel good for a while—it might be months, days, or just a few precious hours—and then it happens all over again. The majority of patients experience all of these distinct stages. But headaches are very individual, so don't be surprised if your headache doesn't follow the "rules." You may skip one or more of these phases. You might get no preheadache symptoms. Instead, your headache arrives like a bolt out of the blue, with no warning. You may immediately bounce back from your migraine the moment you're released from headache pain, while other people need time to recover from an attack. Whatever form your migraine takes, even if it differs from the majority or "norm," consider that as typical for *you*.

What is prodrome?

We know that during migraine, there are physical changes happening inside the brain. Apparently, these minute chemical changes can begin as early as a day prior to the core of the attack, and may result in a variety of signals known as the prodrome. About half of all migraine sufferers report some kind of prodrome experience, but it doesn't fall into any specific pattern. People can have all types of psychological and physical symptoms. Patients often find they have a tremendous appetite, eating any food in sight. Some patients have a tremendous sexual appetite prior to the onset of a headache. Very often prodrome is expressed as an emotional symptom such as elation, almost a euphoria, and lots of energy. Some people feel especially creative during this period. Others become depressed. At first, you may not be aware of the connection between these prodrome feelings and the impending pain. But patients soon learn to recognize the symptoms. They know it's a warning. Then, when that feeling that something "just isn't right" starts, they brace for the next phase of the attack.

If prodrome tells you when pain is on its way, can you head off an attack?

You can if you're lucky. By staying in tune with your body's tiny changes and recognizing them in time, some patients do succeed in stopping the headache in its tracks. By taking medication at the first sign of prodrome, and before the aura or first stab of pain hits, you may be able to abort the headache. Attempts to prevent attacks by taking pain-killers every single day can result in rebound headaches. One of the benefits of prodrome is that it can be used as a timer for your medication, a sort of headache-alert system. Some patients report back that premedicating just before the attack really works and that they don't get the headache. For others, there's no avoiding the pain, and you simply have to treat the headache when it arrives.

Is postdrome that awful, achy feeling I have after a headache is over?

Just as prodrome lets you know that a headache is on its way, postdrome lets you know you'll soon be feeling fine again. Although the phase is not pleasant—with its signature symptoms of exhaustion, sore muscles, foggy head, and emotional roller coaster of highs and lows—postdrome is a welcome sign for migraine sufferers. The tired feeling only lasts for a day or so, and then the pain is over. We think of postdrome as the nervous system crashing. It's wiped out, all the neurons have been busily firing, causing pain and other disturbances. Postdrome is just the body's way of insisting on rest. Sleep is what the body needs to restore itself.

My neck muscles tighten up right before a migraine. Would a good massage at that point head off an attack?

If you can feel the muscles tighten, you're probably experiencing a tension-type headache, described in Chapter 1. These headaches seem to be caused by blood flow problems that originate when muscles tighten up in the scalp, neck, and shoulders. Certainly anything that would help stabilize blood flow, such as acupressure or massage, might prevent or cut down on the severity of an attack. But even in true migraine, which is caused by chemical changes and not muscle contractions, a massage can help. There can still be an achy feeling of sore muscles in your neck and shoulders in migraine; it's a reaction to holding yourself stiffly for hours, in order to prevent the pain that seems to accompany any movement during an attack.

My headaches are sharp and stabbing. My sister says she feels a dull throbbing. Are there different kinds of headache pain?

If you question large numbers of migraineurs, the majority will describe a throbbing pain during their headaches, a pounding that seems to keep time with their heartbeats. That rhythmic throbbing is why migraine was called a vascular headache for so long—because it was thought to have a connection to blood vessels. Some people can actually feel the throbbing with their fingers, by pressing lightly over the temporal artery found in front of the ear. You can do it yourself. Place your second finger in front of your ear. Normally, you might feel a tiny pulse. But with migraine, this artery really begins to pound. The area may feel tender and painful because the artery becomes almost swollen. Sometimes it is so distended so that you can actually *see* it throbbing away. Some people feel throbbing over the eyebrow, in the area called the *orbit*. They experience a pulsation in the branches of the arteries that come from the skull. In either case, the bulk of patients tend to use words like "throbbing," "pulsating," and "pounding" to describe their headache pain. Smaller numbers of patients describe what they call ice pick headaches. These feel like jabs, bolts, and stabs deep in the brain. Unlike the dull-edged, drumbeat aspect of a throbbing pain, these headaches have severe, intense, sharp-edged pain. The pain remains constant during the whole period of the attack. The only good news is that these headaches are often more brief than their pulsating counterparts. Eating ice cream can provoke similar, shorter-lived pains; that's why these are also known as ice cream headaches.

Can the kind of pain I feel indicate the type of headache I have?

The way that you feel headache pain can certainly help determine a diagnosis of one type of headache or another. Cluster headache is accompanied by more of a piercing, knifelike pain. I've heard the description of a nail being bored into the head—a constant, driving pain. People who have migraine tend to describe throbbing. The pain is first severe, then suddenly becomes diminished, severe, then diminished—like the pulsation of a blood vessel or the beating of the heart. That's fairly common. Tension headache, on the other hand, is usually described as a steady pain, but one that never approaches the intensity of cluster headache pain. And then there are people who will complain of a mixture: throbbing alternating with stabbing pain. To make things even more confusing, this pattern would seem to indicate a migraine with clusterlike headache pain as one of its symptoms.

Are migraines always on just one side of the head?

Like nearly all of migraine's symptoms, the headache's unilateral, or one-sided, nature is by no means universal. Often, migraine pain starts on one side, but it can shift to the other side, spread all over the head, or move to a single spot above your eye. It can make its appearance in an area near the ear or jaw, or it may lodge in the back of the head near the base of the skull. In fact, if your pain is always on one side of the head, and it's always the same side, you probably don't have migraine after all, you have cluster headache.

Why do I feel pain in my jaw, eyes, or behind my nose during a headache attack?

There is a reason why pain in your forehead, eyes, jaw, mouth, and sinus area often seems linked. These areas are all serviced by a single nerve, the fifth cranial nerve. So, sometimes the agony in one area is linked to pain in another. This accounts for the fact that many migraine sufferers first consult ophthalmologists, thinking the pain is originating in their eyes, only to be referred to headache specialists after eye examinations reveal no cause for the pain. In other cases, people complain of migraine when they're actually suffering from temporomandibular joint syndrome (TMJ), a painful disorder centered in the joints connecting the jaw to the skull. TMJ's links to migraine are still being debated, and isolating symptoms for diagnosis can be difficult, considering that both disorders share the same cranial nerve path for pain.

My eyelid droops during my attacks. Does that mean I'm having some kind of stroke?

In migraine patients, a drooping eyelid isn't an indication of stroke. Rather, the eyelid symptom is thought to be the result of a weakened nerve. The nerve loses its strength due to the repeated interruptions of its blood supply, a shutdown that is common during headache. Drooped eyelids tend to be more common in cluster headache; 20 to 25 percent of people with chronic cluster or simple cluster headache develop a drooped eyelid on one side after several years with the disorder. Occasionally some migraine patients will complain of a drooped lid, but it's not as noticeable and less common than with cluster headache.

Why does my eye get red when I'm in the middle of an attack?

It's not unusual for some people to get a reddened eye. It's linked to blood flow problems and irritated optic nerves. Symptoms involving the eyes are referred to as ocular symptoms by doctors. This may include a dilated pupil, with the center of the eye opening to its widest capacity, making bright light seem even more unfriendly, or a "pinpoint" pupil, with the center contracting to minute size. The pupil is usually affected in cases where the pain is one-sided, the changes to the eye appearing on the same side as the pain. In truly severe attacks, the eyes can look as bloodshot as the fabled "morning after." They may seem watery, or dry and blurry. Some people report no impact on perception even when their eye is flushed; others have impaired vision, along with the bloodshot appearance, on a sliding scale of severity: everything from a slight bleariness to an extreme reaction to light, even temporary blindness.

Is it unusual to look terribly pale during a headache?

Changes in complexion during migraine are hardly rare, considering that many patients can trace their pain in their faces. In some cases a person's skin appears flushed during migraine, while other patients have a pallor with headache. These opposing types were first described as "red migraine" or "white migraine" by a man named du Bois Reymond, and those terms have stuck. In red migraine, the whole face becomes suffused with blood. In rare cases, the eyes almost seem to bulge out of a beet-red, overheated face. In contrast, a white-migraine sufferer becomes almost pasty during the attack. Even the hands can become pale. Some patients first become flushed, then seem to feel their blood drain away, leaving them pale and shaky. The hands tend to be cold during an episode when paleness is present. Biofeedback can help patients reverse this coldness and pallor of the extremities. Pallor is also connected with nausea and vomiting in migraine. During extensive bouts of nausea, patients may seem almost ghostly, with dark rings around their eyes and sunken cheeks, like victims of some terrible emotional or physical shock. Couple this extreme, deathly pallor with migraineurs' classic pained reaction to bright sunlight, and it's not hard to see how some vampire legends may have started.

During an attack, even my skin hurts. Is that just my imagination?

No, it's not "in your head" it's actually *on* your head. This extreme tenderness may be related to a sudden buildup of fluids in your tissues, a condition called *edema*. Swollen tissues in the face and scalp are very sensitive to pressure, so some people do report that with the headache, their face, temples, neck, or scalp become intensely sensitive.

Does anyone else get specific food cravings during a headache?

Most patients don't get food cravings during headache pain; in fact, they usually experience just the opposite—a total aversion to food. Rather, food cravings generally make an appearance during prodrome or aura, before the pain begins. Often these cravings are for simple carbohydrates and sweets, like cakes and candy. Maybe it's the body's way of storing up the energy it knows it will lose during the vomiting associated with migraine, because the moment a headache strikes, most patients report a sudden loss of appetite. Doctors call this symptom *anorexia*. While patients may feel better if they ingest something, food may seem tasteless. They may throw up simply at the sight of it. Most of my patients don't feel as though they can eat; in fact, they're lucky if they can drink during the headache.

Why do I feel so nauseated when I get a headache?

There's some evidence that the symptoms you feel during the phases of an attack depend on what area of the brain is being irritated at the time. Much of the chemical activity associated with migraine can often be traced to the back of the brain near the nausea or vomiting center. When this area is irritated by the changes that occur in blood vessels or by the chemicals thought to be released during migraine, a person may feel nauseous and vomit. Some patients report other gastrointestinal symptoms, such as gut-wrenching belches, hiccups, or repeated gagging and dry heaves. Unpleasant as these symptoms are, they become even worse because every vomiting session seems to intensify some patients' pain, as their blood vessels throb in sympathy. As the stomach empties, people may experience symptoms of dehydration, too. Drinking as much liquid as you can between attacks of nausea is a smart precaution. For a few people, vomiting signals the end of the attack—the moment they throw up, the pain passes.

I get terrible diarrhea during attacks. Is that related to the migraine or is it something else entirely?

Stomach and bowel upset may be associated with your migraine. As many as 10 percent of patients report diarrhea, an enlarged stomach, cramps, fluid retention, or changes in their bowel movements during migraine. In extreme cases, loss of bowel control can occur. Children are most likely to suffer from all these symptoms, but adults sometimes complain of them as well. In rare patients, stomachache is the only pain the person suffers; no headache pain ever appears. These patients have what's called *abdominal migraine*. Once again, children are the most frequent candidates for this version of migraine. Some doctors dispute the idea that this type of stomach ''headache'' is really migraine at all.

My hearing and balance are affected during my migraine. Is that normal?

Reports of dizziness are common from migraineurs during headache, as are blurred vision and other eye-related problems. These are not the same visual symptoms that you get with aura, but rather a bleariness, dryness, or a sensation of eye strain, even what seems like double vision. It's important to be specific when describing your own feelings of dizziness and eye problems, because they can help measure the severity of an attack. By definition, being "dizzy" means that you feel as though you're actually spinning, or as if the room is revolving around you. Is that what *you* mean when you say you're feeling dizzy? A better description for the sensation you feel might be "light-headed," as though you're walking on eggs. Dizziness, or vertigo, tends to be less common than light-headedness and is a more severe symptom. Analyze your own feelings of giddiness until you can really pinpoint the sensation. When digging down to the root of your symptoms, a conversation with yourself might go like this: "I feel a little dizzy. Wait, what do I mean by dizzy? I mean, I feel light-headed. Then, what do I mean by light-headed? Well, I feel like I'm not walking on firm ground." Choose your words carefully when describing your symptoms, because the more you know about your headache, the more you can do to treat it.

I forget things during my attacks. Is that migraine or Alzheimer's?

The answer to that is two other questions: Is your memory loss getting worse over time and is it present between attacks? If the answer to those questions is no, you are almost certainly suffering from migraine, not Alzheimer's disease. If your symptoms go away for periods of time, that's the critical point in making a diagnosis one way or the other. If your history is of a growing number of symptoms that stick around long after the headache pain has left, and if they seem to get worse and worse, *then* you can worry about something else. Most people with a history of migraine, however, notice that when they get an episode of memory loss or clumsiness, it lasts for just a few hours. They take their medication, feel better, go to sleep, and wake up to find that all symptoms have gone—until the next headache. The key is that, in the interim, they're perfectly normal. So if a patient says she has had this memory-loss symptom for twelve years, every single time she gets the headache, along with a whole host of other symptoms, but in between she's perfectly well, and twelve years later you can't find a thing wrong with her, and her

neurological examination is 100 percent—that's a diagnosis
of migraine.

Why do I act like I'm drunk during an attack?

That happens; people will often feel and act as if they can't
function during a migraine attack. They may not be able to
use one or both hands properly. Some people can't form
words properly. People will say, "When my husband gets a
headache, he's always dropping things and his speech is
slurred. I can't understand what he's saying." Or, "I'm
speaking to my wife on the telephone and suddenly the
words came out strangely, almost like she's having a stroke
or is just plain drunk." There are a whole host of symptoms
that mimic drunkenness or being high: a light-headed feeling,
weakness, dizziness, faintness, eye strain to the point of
blurred vision, and more. As to why it happens, migraine is
a disorder that involves multiple areas of the nervous system.
So, in addition to the head, the rest of the body can become
affected. We believe that minute chemical changes are occurring in parts of the brain that control the areas that aren't
functioning properly during an attack, like the ear and nerves
concerned with equilibrium.

What can I do to lessen the severity of an attack?

Treatment can eliminate or alleviate nearly all of the
symptoms of headache described in this chapter, when the
right combination of options is found. The only problem is
finding that perfect combination, your own "magic bullet."
Prepare yourself for cautious experimentation and some dis-
appointments, then get to work. Somewhere among the advice of doctors, the many forms of medication, the discovery
and elimination of your headache's triggering mechanisms,
and the exploration of alternatives to drug treatment, you're
sure to find ways to cut down on your symptoms or get rid
of them completely. See the related chapters for help in forming your own treatment plan.

What do visual auras look like?

How long have you got? The fact is that aura's visual
manifestations are virtually endless. A look at the many examples of aura drawn by migraine patients looks like a reg-

ular "Who's Who" of art styles: there are Picasso-like renderings of fractured faces and cubist landscapes; pointillistic blends of tiny colored dots; mosaics of squares, triangles, or honeycombs; kaleidoscopic patterns, like tumbled shards of stained glass cutting through a field of normal vision; bold, modernistic wavy lines. There are the classic fortlike zigzags called fortification spectra. Then again, aura can be streams of falling stars, ribbons of curling light and color, twisting distortions of the scenes that seemed ordinary moments ago. People may seem surrounded by waves of brilliant color. Swarms of tiny objects, like bees or ants, can swirl and dive across your field of view. Objects appear to shift, dance, and twirl. Other times, aura takes on a terrifying darkness. A punched-out area appears in the field of vision; people and landscapes disappear into a deep black vortex. Your view of a scene may become abruptly sliced in two, with half the world seeming to drop off into an inky void. Bodily distortion shows up, too. There are many who believe that Alice in Wonderland's stretched-out neck and legs in the famous hallway scene were just a reflection of Lewis Carroll's headache aura, a type of distortion that elongates or shrinks your perception of people's bodies, even your own.

How extreme can these aura "visions" become?

Some patients have almost hallucinogenic visions. One patient I interviewed saw dancing images prior to a headache. She would provide the most florid descriptions of images leaping around, waltzing lights and geometric patterns shooting by. Before the diagnosis of migraine, it was thought that she might be schizophrenic, that she was having hallucinatory delusions. Think how disturbing visions like these could be to someone experiencing them for the first time, especially a child. And what kind of panic might an adult feel, getting aura while driving or speaking in public? One teacher I treated was terribly embarrassed when her aura struck in the classroom and she had to explain her odd reactions to the children. People experiencing aura are beset by questions: Are these images real? Are these spiritual visions? Or are these pictures and "black holes" symptoms of madness, disease, or blindness? Aura can affect people in all kinds of ways, and they react accordingly. They may see it as a frightening curse that stops them dead in their tracks, or as some kind of glorious gift, a wellspring of creative ideas and images, as in the case of the mystic Hildegard of Bingen.

I experienced what I believe to be aura for the first time. Frankly, I'm kind of scared. Why would it happen all of a sudden?

We don't know why aura may come on so suddenly, but it happens often and is no real cause for concern. Migraine with aura and migraine without aura may actually be the same syndrome; for some reason certain areas of the brain suddenly become involved. There can be many reasons for this abrupt shift: changes in the person's hormonal balance, aging, reactions to medication they're taking—both migraine drugs and other medicines—even foods that contain chemicals that upset specific branches in the nervous system. There are a lot of things about migraine we can't explain, and the erratic behavior of aura is one of them.

I feel like I'm going crazy with these visions. Is there a real physical reason behind them?

It's thought that aura is caused by decreased blood flow to the brain. If this interruption in the flow occurs in the part of the brain that's responsible for vision, let's say, you'll get a visual aura. If you get a motor-based aura, like numbness or slurred speech, or a smell-centered olfactory aura, it could then be traced to the part of the brain that controls and picks up signals for that particular "sense."

Can you avoid a headache by taking medication during the aura?

It would seem logical that taking drugs during this phase would head off headache pain before it starts. Unfortunately, this doesn't seem to happen. Even the "wonder-drug" Imitrex doesn't have any effect on the headache when taken during aura. It doesn't seem to affect the aura, either. Some doctors believe it may even be dangerous to treat the headache during aura, since many migraine medicines are vasoconstrictors, which act by cutting down on blood flow. Since aura is caused by restricted blood flow, cutting down the blood supply any further might pose a danger, say physicians. I don't agree with this presumption, but even so, I find it usually doesn't help to take drugs during this phase. Most people prefer to treat the headache itself in the moments right before or right after it arrives.

Is there some way to prevent aura, since it can be so disorienting?

Trying to prevent the aura itself can be something of a lost cause. Aura generally lasts only about forty-five minutes. By the time you recognize the symptom and take the appropriate drug, it's already too late. The aura will probably be gone in the thirty minutes it takes most drugs to work. You don't know whether the aura is going away spontaneously or not; it's very hard to prove that the drug is responsible for an aura's fade-out.

There have been some positive studies, however, on drugs called *vasodilators*, that are derivatives of nitroglycerin. These tests were done by H. G. Wolff, a noted headache researcher in the 1950s. Wolff found that if patients take vasodilators, they could abort the aura. One of these vasodilators is called amylnitrate; it comes in a little perle that can be cracked open. Nitroglycerin is placed under the tongue where it dissolves. Both forms are very potent blood vessel dilators that will work to abort the aura. The trick is, nitroglycerin and similar vasodilators work very rapidly; it's in the circulation within a few minutes.

So why is fighting aura a lost cause? Well, unfortunately, nitroglycerin often drives out aura but causes a headache because it dilates the blood vessels and sends the blood pounding through those arteries. So patients weigh the two. Most headache patients will tell you it's the headache pain that's most disturbing, but some patients will tell you the aura is terrible. These people would rather have the pain of headache than the aura, so they take the nitroglycerin or a derivative. In a few patients, when you stop the aura, the headache is aborted completely. But most of the time, if you treat the aura, people will tell you that it goes away but the headache comes on. So they have to treat the headache afterward.

I can't stand any kind of bright light during an attack. Is that really typical?

Not only is sensitivity to light typical—it's almost essential in making a diagnosis of migraine. It's one of the disorder's most common symptoms, along with headache and nausea. Light sensitivity, or *photophobia*, can range from a mild reaction to a complete aversion to any kind of light. Even the dimmest bulb may seem like an intense, penetrating spotlight to a person with migraine. Light may cause a slight ache behind the eyes or a terrible, blinding pain. Most sufferers retreat to darkened rooms during migraine attacks in response to this symptom. It can begin before the pain arrives and last throughout the attack. Other senses may also become acute: hearing is enhanced in what's called *phonophobia*, so that even a whisper may seem like a scream. The sense of touch can turn abnormally sensitive; soft fabrics start to chafe or seem to weigh a person down. Smell can become affected, too, so that a whiff of perfume or cooking smells set off a bout of nausea and vomiting.

Do other people "smell" things that aren't there during an attack, like cooking odors and gasoline?

You're not alone if you get olfactory aura, or smell-related symptoms during migraine attacks. The scents can be pleasant or noxious. Some people report that their nose runs constantly during aura and even during the headache itself. That's another reason why migraine is sometimes confused with sinus headache.

I notice that certain smells make my migraine attacks worse. Is that just a coincidence?

Smells can exacerbate a headache already in full swing or even suddenly conjure one out of nowhere. Smells can be a trigger for migraine attacks, just as foods, weather patterns, and other environmental changes can signal your brain to bring on the pain. You'll learn more about triggers and other factors that can worsen your attack in the following chapter.

Why do I feel so out of sorts even days after an attack has ended?

That's part of the migraine syndrome known as postdrome. There's a feeling of let down during this phase, which many people find is best helped by simply going to sleep. The nervous system is almost in a state of exhaustion. After this draggy period, people feel terrific. The attack is over and they feel great, even euphoric.

I used to have migraines one right after another. But I've been migraine-free for months now. Are they gone for good?

Don't start counting your chickens just yet. Patients may go a year or more between attacks. In the meantime, it's smart to look around and figure out what might have caused this change in your migraine pattern: Do you have better control over your diet, have you changed your environment, did you cut out some stress factors? If you're in love, laughing a lot, or have achieved a new peak of health, you're taking all the right steps to ensure a decrease in the frequency of your bouts. But don't relax your guard completely. Be ready to recognize the signals of prodrome if they should creep up again or if your old triggers make a reappearance. Then again, if you're over fifty, the change for the better may be permanent, since attacks seem to decline in frequency and severity with age. You just may have seen the last of them.

My headaches always arrive at the same time of day. Is that unusual?

Here again, migraine exhibits its highly individual nature. Some migraine attacks follow a very regular pattern. In the majority of cases, migraine attacks appear first thing in the morning, and are almost as reliable as an alarm clock. Others have a completely random pattern, with headaches appearing at all hours of the day and night. About the only thing people agree on is that migraine attacks tend to show up most often on weekends, with Saturdays being a migraine's favorite day to appear—just another way in which the disorder endears itself to its beleaguered sufferers.

All I want is to lie down in a dark room during an attack. Is my body telling me something?

The body seems to crave darkness during migraine attacks, obviously in response to the eye's unnatural reaction to light during an attack. The body is also asking for rest, because it needs to rally all its resources to deal with the physical toll of migraine. You may also feel the need to lie down simply because your sense of balance is a little iffy during an attack. All these things combine to make it wise to find a dark room and a comfortable bed as soon as possible after the pain hits.

I get really snappy during an attack. Is that a real symptom or just a reaction to the pain?

Mood swings are an almost inevitable symptom of a migraine attack and, in fact, help in its diagnosis. They occur in all phases of the attack. In part, these fits of anger are pure reaction. Patients become so sensitive to light, sounds, and smells that even a dim bulb, faint perfume, or the distant chatter of a child can send them into a frenzy of rage: "Can't you see that's driving me *crazy*?!" Even your sense of touch becomes more focused; the slightest pressure of clothing or sheets may irritate you. It can be impossible to find a comfortable position, so you toss and turn, fidget and complain. The senses become so acute that the slightest trigger can set off a wildly exaggerated reaction, like a suddenly ignited fuse on a stick of dynamite.

This extreme response seems beyond your control—and it is. It's a chemical reaction that can only be restrained with drugs or alternative treatments. These reactions usually become worse the more you push yourself to continue to work or do other activities; you're just burning that fuse hotter and faster. Of course, your family, friends, and co-workers can't see all those brain synapses firing away. All they see are unreasonable responses to normal, everyday pressures. These mood swings and irritability can be the hardest things to explain, and the toughest symptoms for the people around you to handle. That's still another reason you may instinctively seek a quiet, darkened room during an attack—to protect yourself and others from the reactions provoked by these seemingly innocent triggers.

I just want to die during my attacks. Am I the only one who has considered suicide during these moments?

You are not alone in feeling that way. When the pain is at its worse and you know another attack is waiting behind this one, death may seem the only alternative. It's not. There are many alternatives to the pain you're suffering, but the only way to find them is with help—all kinds of help. Find a doctor to help you medicate your migraine. Find a psychologist to help you deal with the depression that's both a chemical symptom of migraine and simply the inevitable result of suffering chronic pain. Look for support groups of other migraine sufferers. You will find people with pain like yours, who will share their stories, treatments, and suggestions with you—along with boundless sympathy. There are groups that can help you find all these services; some are listed in the resource section of this book. They'll refer you to still others. If you're feeling suicidal, do not try to tackle the battle with migraine by yourself. Even if family and friends cannot help you, there are plenty of others who can, and will.

THREE

The Causes of Migraine:
A Biological Short-Circuit

CASE STUDY

Mike needed to know. On his first visit, he told me he needed to know exactly what caused his headaches so he could explain to everyone who doubted him just how this invisible pain could stop someone dead in his tracks. Mike is one of the many male patients in my practice. They are all very unique individuals, but most of them tell a story amazingly similar to Mike's when they reach my office. For years Mike had been troubled by regular cycles of pain. Once or twice a year he would wake before dawn with a one-sided headache, tears welling in one eye, and his nose running. "I know what that means the second I wake up," Mike told me. "I know I'm in for a month of horrible, excruciating pain." That's because Mike gets cluster headaches. His cluster follows a bell-shaped curve: It begins slowly with that morning headache. Then there's a gradual increase in the number of headaches, sometimes as many as ten a day, lasting forty-five minutes at a time. Finally, toward the end of Mike's headache cycle weeks later, the attacks begin to taper off. One morning they're gone. Then eight months later the routine would begin again.

I recognized Mike's symptoms the moment he began describing them. Together we developed a plan to stop the vicious cycle of his cluster headaches using oxygen, which

36

Mike keeps in a tank beside his bed. Along the way, Mike learned about headache and migraine—what causes them and how they are different. We discussed the theories about dilated blood vessels and short-circuiting neurotransmitters in the brain. I explained the latest thinking about serotonin and how it affects the sleep cycle. We looked at diagrams and charts, and I gave Mike advice on what to say to skeptics. He discovered there was no definitive answer to the question of exactly what causes migraine—this week, anyway. But Mike is confident he's learning all he can about his disorder and getting the help he needs. The "invisible pain" doesn't seem quite so invisible anymore.

Someone once said that if our brains were simple enough to understand, we'd be too simple to understand them. That's certainly true in the case of migraine. Like other disorders and diseases of the brain, migraine has so far defied complete understanding. However, some idea of how the brain works—and how migraine affects it—are necessary if you're a headache sufferer. Otherwise, you'll never be able to truly grasp the disorder or manage your treatment effectively.

Just how much do you really need to know? Well, it has been demonstrated that certain forms of migraine therapy, like biofeedback, work better if the patient has some basic knowledge of how migraine impacts the brain. Then you can target the therapy. It's also easier to interpret information you find on migraine if you know the lingo. If you need a refresher course on brain biology, be sure to read these introductory paragraphs before you continue with the chapter. They will give you the basics you need to make sense of the information in this book.

Starting from the top: When referring to your head, what you call skin and bone, a doctor terms *epidermis* and *skull*, or *cranium*. Headache pain can make itself felt in the thin layer of muscle, tissue, and blood vessels sandwiched between your scalp and skull. Lightly press your hand flat against the top of your head, then wiggle your eyebrows. You'll feel muscles shifting under your skin. Lay your hands along the temples and move your jaw as if you're chewing. You'll feel more muscles move. All these muscles tightening up and stiffening are the root of tension headaches.

But we believe that the source of migraine goes much deeper than these surface muscles and tissues, originating inside the skull. That's what doctors mean by *intracranial*. Under the hard bony covering of the cranium, the brain is protected by a layer of "shock absorbers," a thin covering of membranes called the *meninges*. Much of headache's pain originates here. The tough outermost layer of the meninges is the *dura mater*. Below that is the slippery *arachnoid layer*. Then comes the *pia mater*, a very thin tissue made up of tiny blood vessels that cling to the surface of the brain. These vessels are key factors in migraine pain.

The brain itself is largely a mass of gray tissue folded into a rounded lump that fits inside your cranium. Unfolded and flattened, the tissue would cover about three square feet. This brain tissue contains over ten billion cells, or *neurons*, each of which processes hundreds of messages every second, rocketing them from one cell to another at speeds of over 250 miles per hour. As you learn more about migraine's causes, you'll realize how the disorder can affect the way these messages are sent and received.

The brain is made up of many small components, but there are two major players: the *cerebrum* and *cerebellum*. The names are confusingly similar but they perform different roles. The cerebrum—with its bumpy outer layer called the *cerebral cortex*—is the part of the brain you see in horror movies, inching across the floor or pulsating in glass jars. It controls your emotions, thoughts, conscious actions, memory, hearing, speech, and vision. You can imagine how chemical irritants here would cause many of migraine's classic symptoms. The cerebrum has a deep crease running down its center dividing the cerebrum into two perfect halves. These are called *lobes* or, like the halves of the globe, *hemispheres*.

The cerebellum is the other major player. It is nestled under the back of the cerebrum and is about the size of your fist. It controls your physical movements and any muscle groupings that have to work together for complex activities, like the balance needed to climb steps, the hand-eye coordination you need to play tennis, or the instinctive skill it takes to avoid a swerving car on the highway. During migraine attacks, changes in this area are the culprit behind a staggering walk and dizziness. The cerebellum works closely with the nausea and vomiting center of the brain, too.

Tucked up in the middle of your brain is a thick knob on the end of your spinal cord called the *hypothalamus*. It is especially important in migraine. It's in charge of sleep, body temperature, eating patterns, sexual activity, alertness, dreaming, and some emotional responses. You can see why many doctors think some symptoms and triggers of migraine can be traced back to this area. It would explain the way some attacks begin with sexual exertion or changes in sleep patterns and diet, and why your emotional reactions may appear extreme during an attack.

The brain rests on a thick stalk called the *brain stem*, which is filled with nerves. There are twelve cranial nerves conducting messages between the body and brain. These nerves radiate throughout the brain, but all collect into a tight bundle in the brain stem. The stem leads into an area physicians call the *cervical spine*, but most people call the neck. Then the *spinal cord* begins. Is it any wonder that headache, back pain, and neck pain are so closely related, when their nerves are so closely connected?

And, of course, running through this network is blood, supplied to the brain by arteries and blood vessels. This system of blood supply, the *vascular system* or *circulatory system* so often referred to in migraine therapy, is literally the lifeblood of the brain. Unfortunately, it's also an important player in headache pain.

The lesson ends here, but your questions are probably just forming. Hopefully, they'll all be answered in the rest of the chapter. The most important thing to keep in mind is that migraine is a disorder that involves all these complex mechanisms of the brain. While its causes may be the source of heated dispute among doctors, no one denies one striking truth: Although migraine begins in your brain, it's not all in your head. You'll learn why true migraine is considered a primary disorder—the source of your symptoms, not just a sign of something else—and not a psychological one.

What happens to the brain during a migraine?

The question seems simple but the answer can be controversial. Current thought is that migraine begins inside the

brain as a chemical disturbance when something irritates the
brain at a submicroscopic level. No one knows why this
chemical disturbance begins, except that a tendency for it is
inherited and can be kicked off by some outside trigger like
a food you eat or a change in your sleep pattern. This chemical reaction short-circuits the way messages are passed from
neuron to neuron, or cell to cell, inside your brain. This
short-circuit starts off a cascade of events that eventually has
an effect on the blood vessels in your head. These blood
vessels open wider than normal for a time—they *dilate*—
and blood begins to flow in greater amounts. It may even
seem to pulse and pound with the rhythm of your heart. This
sudden, pulsating rush of blood is what's responsible for
some of the headache pain and other migraine symptoms.
The increased blood flow may allow chemicals to leak
through the suddenly thinned shell of the vessel, or the excess blood may aggravate parts of the brain. Doctors aren't
sure exactly what is happening inside the brain during an
attack, but brain scans and other tests reveal that changes,
temporary and tiny, but disabling, are occurring in the brain
tissue.

One doctor says migraine attacks are caused by blood flow; another says it's chemicals in my brain. Which is right?

For years it was thought that migraine attacks were caused
by the flow of excess blood through dilated blood vessels in
the brain and scalp. But now there's good reason to suppose
that migraine begins in the chemicals of the brain's nervous
system, and simply *results* in dilated blood vessels. So a
newer theory is that dilated vessels produce the pain but
don't actually initiate the attack. The two sides of this argument could be called neurological versus vascular, or nervous system versus blood supply. I occupy the third camp
in this medical battle; doctors who think migraine is a combination of the two. We call migraine a *neurovascular disorder*. Our belief is that migraine starts in the brain, but very
rapidly the circulatory system in the brain becomes involved,
sometimes even the rest of the body as well. This theory of
a chemical beginning is supported by the mood swings experienced by migraineurs—a symptom that can't be ex-

plained by increased blood flow, but which makes complete sense when you assume there's a neurological disturbance inside the brain. The sensitivity to light and sound felt during an attack can also be explained this way. Of course, many of the other symptoms felt by sufferers are directly related to the blood vessels widening and other peripheral changes that occur. These symptoms can include cold hands and feet. The fact that many of the medications that successfully fight headache pain work specifically on the blood vessels also makes it clear that there is a tremendous impact on the vascular system, and that there is a relationship between the vascular system, migraine pain, and other symptoms. So we think blood vessels do play an important role in migraine attacks; they're just not their cause.

A lot of this sounds like guesswork. How much do we really know?

Doctors and patients are learning more every day, but granted, a lot of the information collected is hypothetical for now. Obviously, up until now we haven't been able to study someone too closely when he or she is having a headache attack. But the most recent studies use up-to-the-minute technology in brain scans, and the results of those tests lend support to the idea of a chemical reaction, because they have shown that brain changes occur during an attack. They demonstrate changes in blood vessels as well, making the combination theory more and more feasible as time goes by.

What is the blood-brain barrier I hear about in migraine?

If you think of the vascular system as a giant river system of mighty arteries and veins, you would imagine the blood vessels as the smaller tributaries or streams that radiate from those rivers. These little streams get smaller and smaller until they break up into a cluster of even tinier strands call *capillaries*. Capillaries carry oxygen-rich blood from the arteries to the tissues and, when that blood is processed, shuttle it back to the veins. Most exchanges of substances occur at this tiny junction, or what's called the *capillary level*. These capillaries are so thin they allow certain substances to pass through them, like sugar, chemicals, oxygen, and nutrients.

But in the brain there seems to be some kind of built-in obstacle, a protective barrier that shields the brain from substances that could harm it—and, unfortunately, some that could help it. Many substances, including drugs such as antibiotics, can't cross the barrier at this microscopic level. Sometimes patients are forced to get injections directly into the fluid of the spinal canal, just so the medication can get to the brain. If you take the drug peripherally (through the skin)—you inject it into the arm, let's say—it will go through the body but hardly any of it will get into the brain. That's why many medicines aren't effective on a nervous system disorder.

There are exceptions to this rule, but in general there is a barrier at the capillary level. It's thought that maybe the substance molecules are too large to pass through the microscopic openings in the capillaries. A lot of drugs used for migraine don't seem to cross these barriers. So we can assume they are attacking only the extracranial effects of migraine, by helping the blood vessels outside the skull return to their normal flow. Drugs can be effective against extracranial effects such as nausea and vomiting.

What causes the aura?

Unlike migraine pain, which is brought on by an *increase* in blood flow, the aura is thought to be created by a *decrease* in blood flow across the surface of the brain before a headache. This decreased flow is what doctors call *ischemia*. Patients have participated in studies where harmless levels of radioactive substances were traced through the blood, showing us where the flow had been cut down. The results clearly showed a decrease in blood flow during aura, although not to the point where a person will develop a stroke. The kind of aura you get—visions, smells, sounds, disconnected movements, or slurred speech—depends on which area of the brain is losing its supply of blood. Different areas of the brain control different body functions and perceptions.

What is *referred pain*?

The nerves from the spine meet up with the nerves from the face, sinuses, forehead, and ears at a place called the *trigeminocervical nucleus*. Obviously, with all the action going on in the body at any given moment, this area is a boiling cauldron of mixed messages. If your nerves are suddenly irritated, the brain gets confused about where the signal is coming from, especially if it's an acute irritation such as a pain signal. That's why a migraine can feel like sinus pressure, or the stiffness of a back joint can be translated into what seems like a headache. It's similar to the way the brain feels pain and numbness in an arm when someone's having a heart attack. Nerves from those two areas are linked. That's what's meant by *referred pain*, it's simply the brain mixing up the messages from converging nerves. Often, physical exams and tests are the only way to eliminate an unrelated problem and to arrive at a diagnosis of migraine.

Are the causes of tension headache and migraine totally unrelated?

Among doctors who believe that migraine attacks have a chemical origin, there are some who believe that tension headache and migraine are parts of the same disorder: tension headache being the least serious form, at one end of the spectrum; migraine without aura next along the line; and finally, people experiencing aura with migraine at the other end. These doctors regard it all as the same physiological disturbance. Other physicians disagree. They believe that tension headache is simply the result of tense muscles and has no chemical origin. Here again, there's controversy.

Are the causes of cluster headache different from migraine?

The source of cluster headaches is, indeed, slightly different. It's thought that cluster headache is caused by changes that impact a very specific part of the nervous system, the autonomic nervous system. These changes have the most profound impact on the *chemoreceptor*, an organ responsible for processing oxygen into the blood. In cluster headache attacks, one view is that the brain isn't getting its full supply of oxygen, so you can see why the use of pure oxygen is one of the treatments for cluster. Breathing the pure gas may stave off an attack because the patient is artificially receiving the needed oxygen that the chemoreceptor isn't providing, or the chemoreceptor may be less sensitive in people with clus-

ter headache. More and more evidence links cluster headache's impaired oxygen levels to sleep apnea and other
breathing disorders.

What is sleep apnea?

Sleep apnea is a relatively newfound culprit in migraine
disorder. Patients with sleep apnea actually stop breathing
for brief periods during slumber. This erratic breathing pattern can cut down on oxygen levels, causing a condition
called hypoxia. It also reduces the amount of blood flowing
to the brain. Sleep apnea seems to have a relationship with
snoring and is more common in men. This prevalence of
sleep apnea among males may explain why cluster headache,
a disorder that seems to be caused by low oxygen levels, is
also more common in men.

Do the changes in blood flow in my head have an impact on my heart?

No. Although the number of beats per minute may change
very slightly, there's usually no significant change in the
heart's action during a migraine attack. Blood pressure might
go up a little bit, but there aren't any consistent or dramatic
shifts with migraine. The only real vascular impact is on the
width of the blood vessels and the increased sense of pulsation. You may feel this throbbing sensation in your temporal artery, between the eye and ear. Pain-sensitive tissues
around that artery set off impulses that make you aware of
a pounding feeling.

Where's all that blood going?

The blood is going to the head, rushing around and pounding through its countless capillaries. This increased flow to
the brain and surrounding areas may account for the chilled,
bloodless feeling in your hands and feet. The brain is already
the target for 25 percent of the blood in your body; increasing
the flow creates irritations to the tender tissue and nerves
around the brain. And in the nervous system, irritation means
pain.

What is serotonin?

There's a lot of talk in migraine circles about the role of serotonin in migraine. Serotonin is one of the neurochemicals; it controls some of the chemical messages sent from one cell to another. These messages tell the body and brain to perform every conceivable function. Serotonin's particular messages relate to muscle tissue, digestion, and, most importantly in migraine, the cue for blood vessels to contract, or narrow. It's essential to generate this contraction of the vessels in order to curb headache pain. Through microscopic studies we've seen clear-cut changes in serotonin's messages during a migraine attack, so we know by targeting this chemical in migraine treatment we're effectively fighting the disorder.

Serotonin is sometimes also called a *chemical mediator*. It has an impact on other chemicals in the body, such as endorphins. Endorphins are sometimes called natural painkillers, and when released by the body they create a feeling of pleasure. They don't work as well when serotonin levels are disturbed. There are other neurochemicals that may play roles in migraine; one is noradrenaline. Noradrenaline constricts blood vessels and may cause some of aura's symptoms. Bradykinin is a kind of natural *toxin*—or poison—found at the neuron level that aggravates tissues by causing swelling, tenderness, and pain, and also dilates blood vessels.

How does a neurotransmitter work?

The brain is made up of *neurons*, or cells. Each of these neurons collects and passes along information on something happening in the body or mind. They pass these messages along a chain of neurons, like a child playing "telephone," but with much more accuracy. Their "messages" are really chemicals that the brain translates into emotions, thoughts, or sensations: everything from "breathe" and "swallow" to "outrun that mugger" to "love." The neurotransmitter is released from the neuron and it activates an impulse to send a message on to the next neuron, and the next, and so on, getting it to all the necessary brain centers. The neurotransmitter of one cell seems to fit into the receptor on the next cell, or come so close to it that messages can jump the gap between, called a *synapse*. It's believed that migraine pain may originate at this microscopic level. Something goes wrong with the chemical—no one is sure exactly what—and a pain message is signaled to the brain.

I hear a lot about receptors in connection with migraines. What are they?

A receptor is the site where one cell connects with the neurotransmitter of another cell. The receptor is responsible for collecting messages from other neurons. It's ready to accept the chemical message and pass it on.

What do blockers do? And how are they useful to migraineurs?

Called *beta-adrenoceptors*, these, in part, block the receptors that carry messages to dilate the blood vessels. Beta-blockers work on headache pain by shutting off the paths through which that particular message is relayed. They interfere with some chemicals at the neuron level, reducing blood pressure and regulating other aspects of blood flow. Beta-blockers do their trick on the blood vessels outside the brain, never reaching into the brain tissue. They may be working on blood vessels in the heart and other organs as well. More than half of the patients who use beta-blockers find that the number of headaches they get is reduced by 50 percent or more. Beta-blockers never get rid of migraine completely, but they do provide enormous relief when it comes to frequency and severity of attacks.

My doctor told me that the brain can't feel pain. If that's true, why does it feel like someone's drilling into it with a nail?

Your doctor is right; brain tissue can't feel pain. That's why you'll sometimes see films of brain surgeons having casual conversations with the patient whose skull lies open on the operating table. Not only does the brain tissue feel no pain, it can perform many functions while being poked and prodded. There are, however, arteries and blood vessels woven in and around the brain that do feel pain, particularly those in the meninges, the membrane that covers the brain. The pia mater layer there is teeming with blood vessels which are all pain sensitive. You may also be getting signals from the nerves that run into the base of the brain. And, unlike tissue in the brain, tissue cells in your face, neck, and in your scalp are only too pain-sensitive. Other sites around your head that feel pain are the sinuses and muscles. So, the sensation of drilling pain only feels like it's in your brain tissue. It's actually everywhere in your head but there.

What other pain centers besides the ones in my brain are affected by my migraines?

Migraine clearly has a huge impact on both the vascular system and the nervous system. That impact can definitely be felt in more places than just the head. Migraine is a multiple-organ disorder, sending its feelers out all over the body, which explains the tingling in the limbs, numbness in hands and feet, abdominal pain, and chest pain felt by some migraineurs.

Can I inherit migraine from my parents?

The sad news is that migraine does appear to be an inherited disorder. While no one can agree on precisely what sets off an attack, there's one fact that seems certain: The majority of sufferers are predisposed to migraine; it is a genetic trait. In fact, over 60 percent of migraineurs can trace a family history of the problem. They may have an uncle or cousin, father or sister with migraine. But in at least 50 percent of people who have noted a family member with migraine, it's their mothers who have the headaches. You inherit the *tendency* for migraine and then a personal trigger occurs—and a trigger could be any one of a number of things—which sets off your headache.

My mother gets terrible migraine attacks, and I started getting them in my early twenties. Will my son get them, too?

Most migraine researchers agree that migraine can be classified as an *autosomal dominant disorder*, meaning that it can be passed from one generation to the next even if just one parent suffers from chronic headaches. So, yes, your son may suffer from migraine. In fact, studies show that boys are actually more likely than girls to get childhood migraine. But your son may outgrow his headaches, simply because of his gender. These same surveys show that adult men are nearly three times less likely to have migraine than women. Headaches usually disappear in boys as they reach puberty—about the time migraine shows up in girls.

What role do triggers play in the cause of migraine?

Triggers don't cause headaches; they just provoke them. It's a fine distinction that can be difficult to understand. Think of it this way: Migraine is like a man itching for a fight. His aggression, like migraine's, is ingrained. So when his team loses a game, he may take it out on the nearest bystander wearing the wrong team colors. Is the losing team or bystander responsible? No, but they triggered a reaction in someone already primed for it. That's the way migraine triggers work. They don't really cause the attack but simply start the ball rolling, they give an already-primed brain a little push. The brain is primed by genetics; the predisposition is already there. Some outside event, such as stress, a chocolate-eating binge, sudden exertion, or the use of a drug, might be the trigger that sets off an attack. But, just as a fan who takes winning a bit too seriously might do well to avoid no-win games, so must a migraineur learn to avoid triggers that set off an attack.

I'm a very aggressive, goal-oriented person. I've heard that personality may be the problem behind headache pain. Is that really the cause of my migraine attacks?

Years ago you might have been labeled as a *migraine personality*, which was the name some doctors gave patients with particularly driven, ambitious personalities. It was thought that people like this were more likely to get migraine and that these personality traits were the psychological cause of migraine. But more facts have come to light demonstrating what many migraine patients knew instinctively, that their pain is physiological—biological in origin—not psychological. In addition, we've learned through surveys and studies that migraine doesn't discriminate. The disorder strikes people of all different personalities. The real factor in cause is heredity, not personality. Carefree and easygoing people are just as likely as control freaks to get headaches if there's a family history of them. But stress addicts beware. While anxiety brought on by an intense need to succeed may not be the root cause of migraine, it can certainly be a trigger. Just as strong sunlight, traveling through different time zones, and aged cheese, stress can bring on an attack in someone already predisposed to the disorder. Relaxation techniques may be a good alternative for people whose personalities or jobs don't allow them to eliminate the stress trigger from their lives.

What role do hormones play in migraine attacks?

There is a clear link between hormones and migraine. And anything that rocks the balance, or *homeostasis*, of your hormones can trigger the onset of migraine and subsequent attacks. This connection between hormones and migraine has been easier to recognize than many other migraine triggers, primarily because observant female migraineurs have long been able to link their headaches to menstrual cycles, pregnancy, or menopause. Dramatic changes in progesterone and estrogen levels can cause changes in the hypothalamus of the brain, which controls your body's regularly timed functions, such as sleep patterns and menstrual periods.

Can steroids cause migraine attacks?

Any hormonal change can trigger migraine; that includes the use of steroids. Some forms of steroids are used as medication for migraine, to stop headaches already in progress. But nonmedical use of steroids can actually trigger a headache attack—and that's only one of its unpleasant side effects.

What effect do melatonin levels have on migraine?

Melatonin is a natural hormone produced by the body but is now available as an over-the-counter drug in tablet and liquid forms. Melatonin is closely linked to sleep; some patients take melatonin to help them sleep, and the pineal gland produces its highest levels of melatonin during slumber. It may also help keep hormonal balance steady, in homeostasis. Definitive evidence is still unclear, but melatonin may be a factor in migraine. The U.S. Food and Drug Administration is looking into the effects of taking melatonin in over-the-counter form and may make it a controlled substance.

My doctor says my attacks are hemiplegic. I know that has something to do with genetics, but what?

To strengthen the hereditary link, doctors have found that some rare forms of migraine, such as familia hemiplegic migraine, *only* occur when there is a family history of that type of headache. If no one in your family has had it, this type of migraine is not in your future. Hemiplegic attacks affect the movement of the eye and may leave the sufferer with double vision and some temporary paralysis for days or weeks after the headache pain has passed.

Do doctors know which genes cause migraine attacks?

For most migraine types, no specific genetic data is known. With so many recent advances in genetic studies, we may soon know more. But we do think we can track hemiplegic migraine to chromosome 19, one of the twenty-six strands of human DNA.

My doctor says that migraine is a primary disorder. What does that mean?

When migraine is the cause of all your symptoms, it is called the *primary disorder*. It is labeled a *secondary disorder* when the migraine itself is only one of several other symptoms in some other disease or disorder. Then there is migraine as a *concomitant disorder*; that's when you get migraine as a primary disorder at the same time you have another, unrelated primary disorder, such as diabetes. It can be virtually impossible for you to make this distinction yourself, no matter how closely you study your symptoms. Migraine's signals can be too similar to those of other disorders. Therefore, you should go to a physician about your migraine attacks at least once. You can work out nondrug treatments and manage your migraine on your own, but first you have to know what you're fighting.

What other disorders have migraine as a symptom?

Headaches, nausea and vomiting, vision problems, and dizziness: unfortunately these could all be symptoms of many things besides migraine. Migraine can mimic or hide other things that are more dangerous than a headache disorder, so be alert for new or unusual combinations of symptoms. Meningitis, an inflammation of the membranes in the spinal cord and brain, is accompanied by migrainelike symptoms but also features fever and a stiff neck. A cloudy film creeping over the eyeball and a vision of rings around every light source may indicate glaucoma, even if other symptoms like pain around the eye resemble your normal migraine attacks. Glaucoma is not related to migraine, and migraineurs get it no more often than other people; but if you start to get visual symptoms, don't automatically attribute them to your headache. A blow to the head followed by migraine could mean a subdermal hematoma, or blood clot, instead of simply a post-traumatic migraine (a migraine resulting from the blow). Stomach disorders, appendicitis, flu, or stroke are some things you should eliminate as even remote possibilities. High temperatures, seizures, memory loss and confusion, shortness of breath may signal disorders that have migrainelike symptoms. Complacency on the part of patients is okay only if they have been diagnosed, and know they aren't harboring some other illness.

Do severe headaches indicate a brain tumor or aneurysm?

Less than 1 percent of patients can trace their migraine to a brain tumor; it's very rare. Usually, by the time migraine attacks appear as a tumor symptom, other more eye-catching symptoms have already appeared on the scene, such as perception and movement problems, radical personality changes, and slurred speech. While these sometimes accompany headache pain in migraine, in a brain tumor they show up long before headaches begin to make their appearance. Though unlikely, the possibility of a brain tumor can be ruled out by consulting a physician and getting an accurate diagnosis. An aneurysm is a segment of a blood vessel that is weak and has expanded to bursting point, like an overblown balloon. If you experience a sudden, excruciatingly severe attack of pain, more agonizing than any migraine pain you've had before, that's when to check for aneurysm. It's usually accompanied by a stiff neck, fainting spells, and feelings of confusion. This, too, is rare in migraineurs.

What impact does my hypoglycemia have on my migraine attacks?

Hypoglycemia is essentially the flip side of diabetes, but both relate to the levels of sugar in your blood. Blood sugar is broken down by insulin; in diabetics the insulin doesn't perform this process effectively so sugar levels are high; in hypoglycemics, the insulin is too active. The result is low blood sugar. Low blood sugar can be a trigger of migraine. In addition, insulin fluctuations can cause blood vessels to contract and dilate—a source of migraine pain.

What is hypertension? Does it just mean stress?

Hypertension is not the same thing as stress, although stress plays a factor in raising your blood pressure. They're linked, just as stress is clearly linked to migraine. But the connection between hypertension and migraine is not as clear. In order for headache to result from high blood pressure, your blood pressure would have to be incredibly high. That is not common at all. There may appear to be a more direct link for the simple reason that medications taken to treat high blood pressure also have an effect on migraine pain. That's just a lucky break for patients with both.

In order for there to be a connection between your migraine and your blood pressure, for it to be labeled a *hypertension headache*, your pressure would have to experience a very abrupt rise to about 200/130. (A blood pressure measurement consists of two numbers: the higher number is the systolic pressure which is the amount of force, in millimeters, that is exerted by blood on the walls of blood vessels and arteries during heartbeats; the lower number is the diastolic pressure which is the force exerted *between* heartbeats while the heart is resting. A blood pressure reading of 120/80 is generally considered ideal.) It is normal for your blood pressure to be a bit high at the doctor's office, because you may be experiencing "white coat" syndrome, where you are so nervous about the exam itself that your blood pressure goes up during the test. It's best if you rest peacefully for a few minutes or half an hour before you take a blood pressure test, so the stress of seeing your doctor isn't a factor in your levels.

I hit my head in an accident. Can such a blow be responsible for the headaches I've been getting ever since?

Post-traumatic headaches, as these are called, do occur. People may get headaches for months or years after a blow. You should, however, check with doctors to be sure you're not feeling the pressure of a subdermal hematoma, or blood clot. One indication of this is worsening of the pain with each attack.

My headaches have changed since an injury to my head. Is there a connection?

If you have any kind of radical change in your migraine pattern, you should have it checked out. In this case, it could be a blood clot causing the shift in symptoms.

What is TMJ?

Those initials stand for temporomandibular joint syndrome, and you might get it if the joints connecting your jaw and skull aren't aligned properly. This syndrome is often misdiagnosed as migraine. Most specialists feel that it is a distinctly different disorder, though. The areas where TMJ pain is felt are serviced by the same cranial nerve pathway used by nerves feeling headache pain, so the signals can get mixed up. The resulting pain is called *referred pain*.

How are sinus headaches different from regular migraine headaches?

The sinuses are cavities filled with air. They can be found in the bones of your forehead, nose, and cheeks. Normally, sinuses don't "feel" pain; they're insensitive because they're simply holes. But when these holes become filled with fluid or mucus, pressure builds up, and that's when a true sinus headache occurs. But most of the time, this isn't what happens to someone who is diagnosed with sinus headache. What's really going on is a migraine attack. There are blood vessels located near all the sinus points that become dilated during migraine, and the pain is felt in the same areas as sinus headache. Another symptom that makes people think "sinus" is that in cluster headache a patient may get a runny nose on one side. The sinuses aren't blocked, though, so it's not a sinus headache. Contrary to what you see in TV ads, sinus headaches are not that common.

I only get a headache on one side—the side with weaker vision and cataracts. Are these disorders linked?

Yes, they could be linked. Nerves in and around the eye lose strength after years of battling migraine, so weaker vision could result and the damage could be permanent. It isn't definitive, but many patients have noted this relationship.

Is there a relationship between my asthma and my migraine attacks?

Asthma is a result of allergies, which trigger an attack. Allergies may be a contributing factor or trigger in migraine, but so far studies have not shown a clear connection. Certainly antihistamine, taken to relieve some allergy attacks, is known to bring on headaches, since one of its effects is to dilate blood vessels.

My husband started getting migraine attacks after he turned fifty. Is age a factor in the origin of migraine?

There is more likely to be a decrease in migraine attack after the age of fifty, rather than a sudden onset of them. People this age can suffer from migraine mimics such as *temporal arteritis*, an inflammation of the arteries serving the region around the eye. People can start getting migraine attacks at any age, but the number of new sufferers drops off substantially after age forty. So if you've just started getting headaches and are over fifty, you should rule out other disorders before arriving at a diagnosis of migraine.

Can sudden release from stress cause migraine?

Oddly enough, yes. This is sometimes known as a *let-down migraine*. It may be due to the fact that you have been running on high during the stressful time, but once it has ended you let your guard down. And wham! Suddenly the pain appears. It's like cases where parents act on a surge of adrenaline to effortlessly lift cars off children pinned underneath only to feel the torn muscles later. You may react the same way in stressful situations, switching into high gear for a time blocking out other responses. Then the acute crisis is over and the brain opens itself up to other signals, like migraine.

My migraine attack hits every Saturday. What's the cause of chronic weekend headaches?

When you consider that a lot of migraine's action originates in the hypothalamus, and that the hypothalamus controls the body's cycles, the connection becomes clearer. Your body becomes accustomed to a particular sleep pattern during the week, which means going to bed and getting up at routine hours. Once the weekend arrives, people throw their workday routines out the window. They stay up late and sleep in. In someone hereditarily predisposed to migraine, this disruption of the sleep cycle can create a response that results in headache pain. Whether this response is the cause of your migraine or just a trigger is still unclear, but the connection between sleeping late on weekends and headaches is not disputed. Many patients notice it on their own and make the right decision for treatment: They wake up at the same hour on weekends as they do during the week. The weekend headaches usually disappear, or at the very least lessen in frequency and severity. Migraineurs are always wise to maintain the body's status quo.

How can I tell if I'm at risk for migraine?

The only accurate way to know that is to look at your family tree. Does anyone in your family have migraine? If the answer is yes, then you're at risk. But don't just resign yourself. You may not be able to control your genetics, but you can manage your migraine. Look at your lifestyle: Do you have a healthy, well-rounded diet? Do you have ways of dealing with daily stress? Do you avoid caffeine? A look through the next chapter will have you develop a plan for treating your triggers and reducing your risk of getting migraine headaches.

FOUR

The Common Triggers of Migraine

CASE STUDY

During an attack, Rob would bargain with God: "Give me anything else, just take away this pain." But even the pain wasn't as bad as the nausea or the aura. Rob would rush home at the first sign of aura because he was embarrassed by the way he behaved: "I'd stagger around like I was drunk, throwing up, so dizzy I could hardly stand. I had trouble saying simple words. I know people thought I was stoned and that made me crazy." During an attack, the headache pain was intense, and Rob complained of an all-over achy feeling. The day after an attack, he'd wake feeling washed-out and groggy. His headache hangover convinced people that Rob had a drinking problem.

Rob was typical of many of my male patients. It had taken him years to admit he had headaches. He'd used every other excuse in the book to cover his absences from work and postpone activities with friends. He chewed on aspirin until the grinding pain couldn't be ignored. Rob became convinced he had a brain tumor and finally saw a doctor. He insisted on every feasible test and scan, but they all came back negative. Rob still wouldn't admit to having migraine. He thought migraine was something only women got and refused to accept his diagnosis when he first came to the clinic. His attitude changed when I told him that he could expect at least a 60 percent improvement with treatment. The guarantee finally made him willing to listen.

The first thing we did was start a headache diary. Since Rob was not a patient man, his triggers began to show up immediately. His addiction to caffeine was obvious—he drank seven cups of coffee a day. Time-zone travel was another culprit as well as monosodium glutamate (MSG). When he started reading labels, Rob was shocked to discover how many foods contained MSG. By cutting down on these triggers, Rob's headaches were reduced by half in just the first few months. Not long after he started on Imitrex, Rob surpassed the 60 percent improvement goal I promised him. He still doesn't tell many people about his migraine disorder. Fortunately, by maintaining a trigger-free lifestyle, he has less reason to.

Just what are triggers and why are they so important in migraine management? Well, think of your migraine like a sleeping person who is caught in the delicate zone between sleeping and waking. Suddenly an alarm goes off, and the sleeper reacts without thought, bolting upright, pulses pounding. The sleeper would have woken at some point anyway, but the alarm gave the process a powerful kick-start. Migraine triggers work in a way similar to that alarm.

Triggers aren't the root cause of migraine—genetics and minute chemical changes are more common causes—but they do initiate a chain of events in a migraine-prone brain that results in pounding headache pain.

Fortunately, triggers can often be recognized and avoided. So, before you begin exploring the options of medication, try to identify your triggers. Identifying personal triggers should be every migraineur's first step in managing headache, because your headaches can be reduced dramatically by avoiding triggers. Headaches may even be eliminated completely if triggers can be easily removed.

Sometimes finding your triggers is not simple, though, because most are substances or situations that seem harmless: eating a banana, an extra hour of sleep, a sudden wind from the west, even a big helping of spinach may all be triggers. It's only in the migraineur that these take on a sinister role. As you'll learn in this chapter, bright lights, weather changes, fruits, alcohol, allergies, and dozens of other things can trigger an attack. Stress and depression are also key factors that provoke headache pain. If stress or depression is your trigger, learn ways to cope with these problems. Recognizing that these are your triggers doesn't mean you're crazy or that mental illness is causing your migraine attacks. It might, in fact, be just the opposite. Your headache pain might be contributing to your feelings of tension. Migraine may have caused the vicious cycle: headache → stress from dealing with the headache → headache triggered by stress → more stress. Getting help to learn coping strategies can break the cycle and help both problems.

Managing migraine is all about maintaining your brain's delicate balance. Any factor that tips your homeostasis, or balance, has the potential to be a headache trigger. That can mean anything from hormonal changes experienced during menstruation to the food coloring in a piece of candy. Traveling to a different time zone could be a trigger because it disrupts your sleep cycle. However, it's usually some type of food, or chemical found in food. In fact, 25 percent of all migraineurs can trace their pain to particular food triggers. Top foods in order of culpability: alcoholic beverages such as red wine and beer, chocolate, aged cheese, citrus fruit, and coffee.

Triggers directly or indirectly provoke changes in the blood vessels or brain. They may have an effect similar to an electrical charge spreading across the cortex, setting off pain signals as it goes. This is called a *spreading depression* in migraine. But the truth is, no one is sure what a trigger's exact mechanism is. All we do know is that migraineurs are supersensitive to chemicals that do not affect most people, and are incredibly attuned to environmental changes. Apparently your trigger develops when your brain becomes particularly irritated by one of these chemicals or changes. After the first encounter, the irritating factor automatically provokes the same response every time it appears: pain. Headache is just the body's emphatic way of saying "Stay away from that!"

So, do what your body's telling you. Stay away! A simple change in diet or lifestyle can go a long way toward eliminating your headaches. Of course, it's not always easy to do that. And sometimes you may even feel that splurging on something is worth the hours of pain you know will follow.

After all, who would turn down a trip to Paris even if air travel is a trigger? Dealing with triggers involves avoiding them when you can and using measures to alleviate the inevitable pain when you can't.

In some cases a trigger is virtually unavoidable. Strong sunlight is a common example. Some sufferers simply shrug their shoulders and accept the pain. Don't settle for that. If you can't eliminate a trigger, control your reaction to it. Try biofeedback, hypnotism, and the other alternatives described later in the book. Explore the options of drug therapy with your doctor. Test yourself to see how the trigger works in combination with other factors that *can* be avoided.

In other cases, it may not be sensible to eliminate triggers completely. For instance, no one should cut citrus fruits or important vegetables out of their diet without experimenting to see how much can be eaten without provoking a headache. Moderation is the word to remember. Find out how much of your trigger you can handle before it acts as an alarm for headache. Learn your threshold and respect it, and you'll be taking control of your migraine.

How can I identify my triggers?

Trial and error is the key to identifying triggers. If you already have some idea of yours, that gives you a head start. Look up your suspects in the chart on page 197. Are your triggers listed there? If you know that a certain prepared food provokes your headache, check its ingredients against the chart, too. Today, all foods must provide nutritional and ingredient lists in a standard form that makes it easy to spot potential triggers like monosodium glutamate or high levels of sodium. If you haven't a clue what your triggers are, there are ways to figure them out. All it takes is some detective work. Start by keeping a headache diary or calendar. Note each attack as it occurs and record the nature and amount of any food ingested in the hours prior to the migraine. Try to recall the circumstances and environment in which the trigger could have been. Why is that important? Studies show that some triggers work only when taken in certain amounts or in a specific situation. You may discover, for instance, that your red wine migraine attacks appear only after a second glass, or when you drink at stressful business functions.

Sticking to only one drink or sipping only in more casual conditions may disarm that trigger. So try to recall where you'd been, what the weather was like, and what your emotional state was in the hours prior to an attack. If no patterns emerge after a few months, you may have to try an elimination diet.

My doctor suggested that I go on an elimination diet to find my trigger. What is that?

The idea behind an elimination diet is that you remove all potential food triggers from your menu until you're headache-free, then begin reintroducing them one by one. In that way, your trigger should stand out like a sore thumb. An elimination diet isn't fun—weaning yourself from addictive triggers beforehand is hard, and the first few weeks offer a pretty bland menu—but it is very effective in targeting your triggers.

You start by eliminating three of the most common triggers from your diet and lifestyle: smoking, alcohol, and caffeine. For those addicted to these substances, this first step is by far the most difficult. Use whatever support and methods you can to wean yourself from these three triggers. You may be rewarded instantly: Perhaps your headaches will stop as soon as you've gone cold turkey. In that case, you may have identified your triggers.

If not, begin the food portion of the diet after you've managed a full week without smoking, alcohol, caffeine, or their withdrawal symptoms—which may include headaches. For the first stage of the diet, your menu should be limited to brown rice, noncitrus fruits, steamed vegetables, and decaffeinated tea. Drink lots of water, too, at least sixty-four ounces a day. Stick with these foods until you've been headache-free for a week (or longer if your headaches occur less frequently than once a week). Then, slowly introduce each trigger food, no more than one a day, keeping track of what you're eating each day. See which foods set off your headache alarm. Start by reintroducing the more basic food staples, like dairy, bread, and fruit. Follow those with processed meats and prepared foods like soups, frozen dinners, and premade sauces. If a food provokes migraine, immediately remove it from your diet once again. Bring it back after about a week to see if you get the same results. If not, consider what else was happening when you ate it that first time: Were you under stress, traveling, or were there changes in the weather that day? Try reintroducing the food a few times to be sure you have found the right trigger.

How long can it take to identify a potential trigger?

Luckily, many triggers are fairly obvious. Some headache patients figure out what their triggers are on their own; they notice a pattern without the aid of a doctor or specialist. Other triggers can be less obvious and take longer to spot, such as minerals and certain chemicals like food additives. You realize how daunting the task may be when you learn that three thousand different chemicals are added to foods to enhance flavor, texture, or color. Then there are the twelve thousand indirect additives that could be introduced into foods through the packaging and manufacturing process, like aluminum from cans and dioxin from milk cartons. So don't be discouraged if finding your trigger takes time. It may take months, a year, or longer to discover what your body's alarms may be, especially if your migraine attacks are infrequent. Don't give up. Keep looking. You'll be rewarded by relief in the end.

If I cut that one thing out of my life, will my headaches just go away?

If you've spotted a trigger and take steps to avoid it, you'll see a dramatic decrease in the number of headaches you get and in the level of pain you experience during an attack. Your migraine attacks may not vanish completely, but you should notice a real difference. A few patients do find complete relief.

If something is a trigger for me, is that the same as saying I'm allergic to it?

That's a good question—so good that it's been keeping people who study migraine busy for years. So far no one has the answer, and there is much controversy over the suggestions doctors have made about possible connections between migraine and allergies. There seems to be a link but exactly what kind is unclear.

Put simply, allergies are the result of your body's reaction to a certain substance. Your body may react to this substance, or allergen, by attacking it with an array of weapons from your immune system arsenal. It's these weapons warring through your body, not the allergen itself, that cause the nasal congestion, pressure, and pain of allergies. This chemical reaction seems similar to the automatic response your body has to migraine triggers.

One of the substances your body produces to fight allergens is called *histamine*. Histamine dilates the blood vessels, causing blood flow to increase and produces *prostaglandins*, chemicals that also dilate blood vessels. Is histamine a culprit in migraine, too? That's still unknown. While antihistamines are usually not effective in treating migraine, some cluster headache sufferers are treated successfully with histamine desensitization. In any case, migraineurs are certainly more sensitive to histamine, so try to avoid that trigger. Besides being produced by your body, histamine can be introduced through foods that contain *tyramine*, another trigger found in red wine, pickled cabbage, sausages, and cheese. Another thing that makes it hard to figure out the migraine-allergy connection is the fact that many people with severe allergies are under stress; it's a chronic condition that's hard to deal with. So the emotional strain brought on by allergies may be acting as a trigger for migraine.

Is emotional stress the cause of my headaches or just a trigger?

It's a trigger. You've heard it before, but it doesn't hurt to hear it again. Your migraine has physiological origins; these changes can be triggered by chemical reactions in your brain caused by extreme emotional states just as they can be triggered by chemicals in foods. It has been noted that serotonin plays a role in both migraine and depression.

Some doctors postulate a genetic connection between emotional stress and migraine. They think that people who inherit migraine may also inherit a depressive gene, and that perhaps these two are linked. It's still very theoretical. Meanwhile, patients experience the classic chicken or egg dilemma: Does the stress trigger the migraine or does the migraine bring on the stress? Like so many things, it's a bit of both. Stress from work may trigger an attack. Then the guilt brought on by facing your family with *"another* headache" triggers more stress. You have to break the cycle by practicing biofeedback and other relaxation techniques or getting drug therapy if you need it.

What are some foods that could be triggers?

Look at the chart on page 197 for a comprehensive listing of trigger foods, then refer to this chapter about why and how they work. Foods, activities, and environment—they can all be triggers.

What is tyramine?

Tyramine is an amino acid, or *amine*, a substance we get from the protein in foods. Tyramine produces adrenaline and affects blood pressure. More evidence is needed to confirm its role in migraine, but it seems that large amounts can cause headache attacks because of its effect on blood vessels. Or perhaps it isn't an increase in tyramine at all, but just a migraineur's sensitive system overreacting to normal amounts. Tyramine is found in sauerkraut, aged cheeses, processed meats such as salami, beer, and aged wine. Some foods, like liver and fish, don't start off with high levels of tyramine, but they start accumulating it as freshness fades.

Does the *amount* of alcohol I drink have anything to do with migraine? Or just *what* I drink, like red wine?

Both can affect migraine. Many patients get their headaches only after a second glass of liquor. Oddly enough, it's not the alcohol that is the trigger, but other chemicals found in some alcoholic beverages. This distinction becomes more apparent when you realize that high-alcohol-content drinks like vodka and gin don't seem to precipitate attacks, while two glasses of red wine or beer immediately introduce a headache. Why? Some people think it's the coloring agents in darker liquors that are behind headache pain. Sulfites used to preserve wine seem to have a connection to migraine, too.

To cut down on wine-induced attacks, stick with one glass of wine, switch to light-colored liquors, and avoid the especially trigger-prone Chianti, sherry, and sauternes. Pay attention to the situations in which your alcohol trigger affects you. Maybe it's only a threat when you drink in stressful situations, like a business dinner or a first date.

I recently switched to a vegetarian diet that includes lots of fruits. Is there any connection to my recurring headache?

Sometimes even good health has its drawbacks. For instance, citrus fruits such as grapefruit, oranges, lemons, tangerines, pineapple, and limes—healthy for you in so many ways—can be triggers for migraine. Nitrogen in these fruits may impact on blood vessels in a way that provokes an attack. Some other staples in vegetarian diets can be triggers, too, like passionfruit, fava beans, spinach, lima beans, lentils, bananas, kiwi, mangos, red plums, papaya, corn, and eggplant. Strawberries contain peptides, by-products of the digestive process that may be triggers; pineapple and papaya have enzymes that may cause an allergy-type reaction that also causes headaches.

Because these foods can be beneficial to your body in some ways, experiment with smaller amounts than you normally eat before cutting them out of your diet completely. Doctors recommend limiting yourself to half-cup servings of these items. There are fruits that you don't have to limit, though, so base your vegetarian diet on them: pears, apples, prunes, cherries, grapes, apricots, and peaches.

What about bread? I heard I can't eat it because of the yeast; is that true?

The trigger here is actually a yeast extract found only in hot homemade breads, sourdough, and breads or crackers made with aged cheese. Let your homemade bread cool and the risk of headache is reduced. Other grain-based products are fine, too, unless brewer's yeast is listed in the ingredients, or if they contain dried fruits like bananas, raspberries, and pineapple, like some breakfast cereals.

Why is salt a trigger? Is it because of its role in high blood pressure?

Sodium is a mineral and it's the main ingredient (40 percent) in table salt. Normally, adults should limit sodium intake to between 1,800 and 2,000 milligrams daily. Before you get excited about that high number, check out the label on a can of soup: One popular brand of creamed mushroom soup has 820 milligrams of sodium per serving. Some doctors think that even 1,800 milligrams is too high, and for supersensitive migraineurs a much smaller amount may be too much.

In high volumes, sodium causes a condition known as *edema*, which is an excess of fluid around some cells. That has an impact on blood pressure rate. High blood pressure is very rarely the cause of migraine, but there may be a salt-related circulatory system connection. Or perhaps it's simply that salt causes dehydration, another common trigger.

I get migraines whenever I'm at the movies. Is it the big screen or the buttered popcorn?

It may be both. There is a lot of salt in the popcorn found in most theaters, and it can dehydrate you if you're not careful. If you drink soda to rehydrate, the caffeine in many colas may act as a trigger, too. Changing light patterns is another trigger you face at the movies. Films contain scenes of highly contrasting images and light. You can see how a trip to the movies can be a migraine waiting to happen. If you know you're prone to headaches when you go to films, don't buy that tub of popcorn, and take some preventive medication beforehand.

Is caffeine in coffee a cure or a trigger? I've heard both opinions.

Caffeine is an alkaloid, a substance that acts as a stimulant. Caffeine is a mildly addictive drug that stimulates the nervous system, heart, and lung action. It also puts the squeeze on blood vessels and opens airways so there's more oxygen supply to the brain, which is why it can be so effective in headache treatment. You can find caffeine in coffee, tea, chocolate, and many colas. Caffeine only acts as a migraine trigger when people are getting too much of it. People may down several cups of coffee a day, supplement it with a chocolate bar or bowl of chocolate ice cream, then have tea or cola later, which contain even more caffeine. Caffeine's normal action of squeezing blood vessels shut is reversed when too much is taken, and the vessels dilate, causing headache pain. Like other migraine treatments, an occasional dose is okay, but when you overuse it, you get into trouble with a rebound headache. That's why caffeine has something of a bad reputation.

Though, like other drugs, harmful when abused, caffeine can be very effective when used in the correct amounts. In addition to its effects on blood flow and oxygen supply, caffeine is known to speed the action of many medicines, migraine drugs included. So it diminishes your pain by enhancing the real painkiller. If you took caffeine alone you might not get much of an effect, but if you take it with an analgesic medication, it could really alleviate your pain. One more note of warning, though: People who suddenly give up caffeine can get withdrawal headaches, so cut back gradually if you're a heavy user.

I seem to get migraine attacks every time I eat chocolate. Is this a coincidence? (Please say yes!)

Unfortunately, the answer is no, it isn't a coincidence. This may be due to the caffeine, theobromides (bitter alkaloids), peptides, or phenylethylamine (an amine that works on blood vessels), found in cocoa. But if you're a chocolate nut, that doesn't mean you have to cut it out of your life completely. By keeping a headache diary you can see what amounts you can consume before a migraine makes an appearance. See if chocolate only acts as a trigger when you eat it at work or in the sun or if you eat a bar with nuts, which is another known trigger. It may be a combination of factors that make chocolate a trigger.

Your headache diary may also shed light on an interesting dilemma facing those with a chocolate trigger. Many migraineurs report a craving for chocolate immediately before experiencing an attack. This poses the question: Does the candy precipitate the attack, or is it merely coincidental to a headache already in progress? Experiment by giving in to the craving some times and holding out at other times. Does the headache make an appearance anyway? A detailed diary may help you determine chocolate's role in your own migraine attacks.

What is the connection between migraine and aspartame?

Aspartame is an artificial sweetener made up of two amino acids, aspartic acid and phenylalanine. It's found in the sugar substitutes NutraSweet and Equal, and is an ingredient in some low-calorie or dietetic prepared foods and drinks. So far, no research has been able to show a definite link between aspartame and migraine. However, because so many patients have noted a relationship and have seen real improvement when they eliminated aspartame, it seems that some connection must exist. It may be worth a try in your own trigger testing. Some medical research shows conflicting results with aspartame in migraine subjects.

Everyone says that MSG (monosodium glutamate) triggers migraine attacks. Is that true?

A connection hasn't been proven by research. Patients and doctors believe there is a link, though, because so many people reduce their headaches when they eliminate MSG from their diets. Chinese food is not the only kind of food that includes this flavor enhancer. MSG is used in frozen dinners, prepared sauces, canned soups and broth, bouillon cubes, textured soy protein, gravy mixes, potato chips, smoke flavoring, dried soup mixes, some processed meats, salad dressings, and some spices. If you look through the ingredient lists of these foods in your grocery store, you'll find monosodium glutamate. Diet meals may include it because they've had to cut back on other flavorful ingredients like salt, fat, and sugars. In some ingredient lists MSG appears as hydrolyzed plant protein (HPP) or hydrolyzed vegetable protein (HVP). Other places where it may turn up is in bottles labeled as "seasoned salt." If MSG is your trigger, read the fine print.

I ordered from a non-MSG Chinese restaurant but got a headache anyway. Why?

Chefs may not consciously add MSG to their dishes, but that doesn't mean it may not be entering your food through less obvious means. When they made their "No MSG" pledge, the cooks at your restaurant may not have realized that MSG is an ingredient in *other* ingredients. Monosodium glutamate can crop up in premade soups used as the base for a dish, vegetable proteins used in place of meat, soy sauce, and other special sauces added to your dish.

I'm trying to lose weight by eating low-calorie foods and skipping meals. Is it a coincidence that my migraines got worse when I started my diet?

There is never an easy "out" when it comes to weight loss. Both diet approaches you named can be migraine triggers. Many low-calorie foods, especially diet drinks, contain large amounts of sugar substitutes. One of the most common, aspartame, may be linked to migraine. Disrupting your normal meal pattern can lead to headaches, too.

In addition to the nutritional problems that lack of food may provoke, skipped meals can throw off your body's meal "clock" and trigger a migraine. The periodicity, or timing, of food intake is controlled by a part of your brain called the *hypothalamus*. Just as the hypothalamus controls the timing of many functions, it also has an impact on the headache sequence. So the key to reducing headaches may be as simple as eating three meals a day. Don't skip meals to lose weight; learn to control your food intake in the same way you're learning to manage your migraine.

My "hunger" headaches don't always go away even after I've eaten. Is there something else triggering the headache?

What you're experiencing still may be migraine. The interruption in your eating routine started migraine's chemical cascade rolling. It won't necessarily stop just because you've eaten; the trigger has already taken effect. When that happens, it may be too late for preventive measures. Now you have to treat the headache itself.

My doctor told me my migraine attacks might be due to low magnesium levels. Can that really trigger headaches?

It's difficult to be sure because so few large-scale studies have been done. However, scattered studies and word-of-mouth evidence supports the idea that the two are linked. How? Magnesium is a mineral present in every one of your body's cells and in unprocessed food, such as some fruits, nuts, beans and other members of the legume family, whole unmixed grains found in cereals with minimal processing, fish, and green vegetables. Magnesium is important in the maintenance of your electrical nerves and muscle cells. Low magnesium levels affect blood vessels and play a role in how efficiently your body uses serotonin receptors. Deficiency can also bring on nausea, weakness, and emotional upset. According to nutritional standards, men should take in about 350 milligrams of magnesium daily, while a woman's RDA (recommended daily allowance) is 280.

But taking over-the-counter magnesium supplements may not help your migraine. In the studies that showed patients improving when they took the mineral, injections of magnesium sulfate were used, not pills. Not much is known about the effectiveness of oral over-the-counter magnesium. The tablets that are absorbed best by your body cost quite a bit more than the others, so patients may not choose them. The brands that aren't absorbed well can cause diarrhea. The vitamin complex B_6 may help in the absorption of magnesium and speed its actions in the body.

It's interesting to note that some doctors think low levels of magnesium aren't just a trigger, but one of the root causes of migraine. They believe these low levels cause the trigeminal nerve to release *peptides*, tiny protein molecules that dilate blood vessels.

Okay, I had some chocolate. I couldn't help myself. Now what do I do?

The goal is to take control of your migraine, but you're only human. Don't beat yourself up if you succumb to a seductive trigger. If eliminating the trigger makes you almost as miserable as the headaches, try experimenting with smaller amounts of it. And when you do use or expose yourself to a trigger, take preventive medication before the pain begins. If you're too late and an attack is already in full swing, try one of the alternative therapies or medications from your treatment plan.

I just discovered red dye #40 can be a trigger. What kinds of foods use the dye?

Food colorings have been plagued by health concerns for decades. As a matter of fact, only about thirty-three are approved by the Food and Drug Administration (FDA) for use in the United States, red dye #40 among them. But having that approval doesn't mean they're healthy for migraineurs. Food colorings are added to make food look better, but they can cause a headache reaction. Yellow dye #5 has also been connected with headache. It has been banned in some countries, although it is still used here. Look for both dyes in the ingredient lists of candies, soft drinks, ice cream, and a range of processed foods that have been canned or cured.

Sulfites, nitrites, and nitrates—what role do they play in migraine?

Sodium nitrite and nitrates are preservatives. In meats, they stop the spoiling process that can cause botulism. Unfortunately, they're also triggers. Some people even refer to headaches triggered by nitrates as "hot dog headaches." Look for these preservatives in sausages, pepperoni, hot dogs, bacon, bologna, ham, liverwurst, beef jerky, corned beef, pastrami, smoked fish, Spam, pork and beans, and other cured meat products. For a migraineur, fresh meats are a safer bet; the aged, canned, cured, or processed meats are what you need to avoid. Sulfites are preservatives, too, used in red wine.

Can a fragrance be a trigger?

Scent is a common trigger. Good smells, bad smells—there is no real pattern. Strong odors are especially likely to provoke headaches. Many migraineurs get an attack after a visit to a gasoline station or exposure to paint fumes. The nose contains the olfactory nerves that transmit impulses to the primary part of the brain and upset the balance in the nervous system of susceptible patients, and this may result in a severe migraine attack. Some migraine sufferers curiously report strange or common odors as aura symptoms.

Yesterday it seemed like the perfume on a woman twenty feet away set me off. Can my migraines possibly be that sensitive to a trigger?

Like the heroes from a comic book, it seems as if migraineurs are superhuman in their sensitivity to sensory signals. The results of this "superpower" are less heroic than those that appear in the comics, however; they bring on migraine attacks. It may take only the barest drift of fragrance to set off a headache. If you usually get headaches in crowded places and can't figure out why, it may be that you've smelled something so distant that you didn't consciously make the connection, but the chemicals in your brain went berserk.

Are foods and smells the only triggers?

Foods and scents are only the tip of the trigger iceberg, as you'll see on the chart of migraine triggers appearing on page 197. Head trauma is another trigger. But far more common triggers include: change in sleep patterns, menstruation, birth control pills, menopause, estrogen pills, drugs, withdrawal from drugs, excessive heat, weather changes (particularly those that make joints swell), stress, depression, letdown after stress is lifted, pressure on certain points of the head, exertion, sex, sunlight, and loud noises. There's also dehydration, bright sunlight, computer monitors, airplane travel, traveling across time zones, altitude, motion, hunger, and environmental factors like pollution. There are so many that it would be impossible to avoid at least one.

Whenever I work in my garden I get a migraine. Could it just be allergies?

It could be allergies, or migraine, or both. Perhaps in your case an allergic reaction to a plant is the culprit, but it could be a combination of migraine triggers: sunlight, fragrance, dehydration, exertion. Note what you're doing and the surrounding conditions when you get your gardening headache. Does it only appear on very sunny days? Do you get it after you've spent hours outdoors without water handy? Does it only show up on days you're hauling weeds and turning over heavy shovelfuls of dirt, and not on days you're performing less physically taxing gardening chores? Does it only happen when you're spraying pesticides or using some other gardening chemical? Are you in the vegetable patch when it comes on, or pulling weeds in your highly scented flower and herb plot?

I get headaches whenever I'm in bright sunlight. Can I do anything to stop that cycle besides wearing hats and sunglasses?

Sunlight is a common headache trigger. Even filtered sun can trigger migraine—patterns from sunlight coming through venetian blinds can set it off, as can other light sources and patterns such as the flickering sparks from a disco ball. You've already identified the two best ways to deal with a sunshine trigger, besides taking preventive medication when you know you can't avoid glaring sun exposure. Other preventive measures are avoiding water and snow sports that involve glare-filled situations.

My headaches seem tied to the length of time there's daylight. Is there a connection?

Some people do report a connection between their headaches and the hours of daylight. This particular trigger seems to show up more in cluster headache patients. In studies, these patients had more headache cycles in January and July—in the week or so after the shortest and longest days. It may be that these periods have an impact on the pattern of your body's internal clock, called your *circadian rhythm*.

Why do I get headaches when I visit my sister in the city?

There could be a number of triggers responsible for headaches that follow a trip to the city, such as increased levels of pollution and noise or the glare off cars, reflective skyscrapers, store windows, etc. Other trip-related triggers may play a part as well, such as the stress of preparing and taking the trip, traveling in an airplane, time-zone changes, trouble sleeping in unfamiliar beds, and less attention paid to avoiding food triggers when you're having a good time. It may actually be the good time itself that's the trigger. Release from the stress of work can cause headaches, called letdown headaches, which explains the pain so many migraineurs experience while on vacation.

It's not as bad as it sounds, however. If you know you're prone to headaches in that situation, there are steps you can take to block all these triggers: everything from using relaxation techniques, bringing a water bottle on flights, wearing earplugs, and requesting a better mattress, to taking preventive medications.

My daughter recently started smoking. That's when her migraine attacks began. Any connection?

Yes, cigarette smoking appears to be a powerful trigger and is a special problem for women. The mechanism behind this is still not clear. It may be as simple as carbon monoxide interfering with the supply of oxygen to the brain. There is a clear link, though, so reducing migraine attacks can be added to the many excellent reasons to quit.

When I've been working on the computer all day, I get migraine attacks. Is it eye strain or something else?

It may be eye strain causing your headaches, or the monitor's flickering screen may trigger an attack. Although they may appear to be steady beacons, most monitors have irregular light patterns, like the pineapple of a disco ball. Migraineurs are very sensitive to any changes in light.

My migraine attacks started occurring in the weeks after moving from sea level to a much higher altitude. Any connection?

Altitude changes can upset the brain's delicate balance, just like any other extreme change. While your breathing seems to adapt quickly, struggle continues taking place in your body. You may still be getting less oxygen than your brain is used to receiving. Try exercising in moderation to increase oxygen intake. There are also prescription medications that can help. It takes several days to acclimate to higher altitudes. It is advisable to avoid alcohol at the beginning of a high-altitude trip.

Why do I get headaches every time I travel by plane?

It may be that dehydration is the real culprit here. The dry air inside an airplane can cause dehydration, even on short trips. Bring your own bottle of water for the period between boarding and the arrival of the beverage cart. And when the cart comes, refuse any alcoholic beverages, which have even more of an impact in high altitudes and can contribute to dehydration. Altitude extremes can trigger headache, too.

However, sometimes it's not the airplane trip itself but the time-zone switch. Travel between time zones irritates the brain center that controls your body's various "clocks," triggering migraine. Jet lag at the end of the trip doesn't help your migraine, either.

Can a drug I'm taking for another disorder act as a trigger?

Some medications used for treating other disorders have headache side effects. You should certainly take a look at any drug you're using when seeking your trigger. Nitroglycerin (used to treat angina pectoris) and certain drugs used to treat hypertension can provoke headaches—even painkillers and antiarthritis medications like indomethacin. Dependence on or abuse of a drug—or withdrawal from one—are conditions that trigger migraine.

My migraine attacks go away if I get really angry. My sister's migraine attacks start when she's mad. How can you explain this?

Adrenaline and other substances may be produced in greater amounts by your body when you're enraged. Like any other change, these increased levels could affect migraine. For some people, it tips the brain's delicate homeostasis out of balance; in other cases, this adrenaline surge may help restore the balance of a brain that has already been disturbed.

This sounds crazy, but I get headaches whenever I have sex. What's going on?

That doesn't sound crazy. It sounds like the complaint of many migraineurs, all of whom are suffering from a condition called *benign orgasmic cephalgia*. It's also sometimes called an exertion headache. Exertion of any kind is often seen as a trigger, or an enhancer that makes pain worse during an attack. The attacks are generally briefer than most migraine attacks, and feature more of a stabbing pain. Cluster sufferers are more likely to have this trigger. For some, the exertion trigger is exercise rather than sex. Even the strain of a coughing fit, sneezing attack, or the strain of a difficult bowel movement may bring one on. Lifting something heavy and having sex are more common triggers, however.

Migraineurs aren't the only people who get a crushing headache that begins with climax; they're just more likely than nonmigraineurs to get one. Tightening muscles in the neck and shoulders may be the triggering mechanism, or it could be chemical in origin. Luckily, taking an ergotamine or beta-blocker such as Inderal or indomethacin before sex can stop an attack before it arrives. With preventive medication and relaxation techniques, there are ways to avoid this pain.

Whenever I oversleep, I wake up with a headache. Is it migraine?

Sleeping problems and disturbances are major migraine triggers. You may require less sleep than other people you know, but everyone needs at least four to five hours each day to recharge your body's and brain's batteries. Your brain has a neurological clock that controls these periods of sleep. When you don't get enough sleep (*insomnia*) or get too much of it (*hypersomnia*), or if your breathing falters during that period (*sleep apnea*), or if your dream state is especially active, your neurological systems become unbalanced. Be consistent in the number of hours you sleep: Variability is what throws off your brain's balance.

Another reason sleep problems may be triggers is that your body controls basic functions differently when asleep, especially when dreaming. It becomes less focused on body function. Body temperatures become more influenced by outside environment, and breathing is less regular. Both factors may contribute to migraine as triggers.

How does dreaming affect migraine?

Any brain activity that happens while you're awake or asleep is centered in the brain stem, which connects the brain to the spinal cord. During sleep, the brain doesn't switch off; it just modifies its activity, which we can record with special sensors. What we know about the stages of sleep, we learned through tracing the patterns of brain waves, which are measured by those sensors. These signal patterns are electroencephalograms, more commonly called EEG. Waves generated by the brain during waking hours are alpha waves. During sleep stages, these waves change. Sleep stage one lasts for only minutes or seconds, and shows half as many wave cycles per second as in waking. These are called *theta waves*. In stage two, the waves become pointy peaks, called *sleep spindles*. Stage three begins when these spindles are joined by slower waves, called *delta waves*. In stage four, delta waves have taken over. These four sleep stages are very smooth and gradual; you repeat the four-stage series many times during the night. In between each series are other stages where you nearly emerge from sleep. These are the dreaming stages, also called REM for the rapid eye movements that signal it, or D-sleep for dreaming sleep. Most sensory perception is blocked and major muscle groups are switched off during REM stage. We become "paralyzed" for our own protection, so we can't act out our dreams. Other functions remain on during REM but become more erratic than when we're awake: Blood pressure and respiration may fluctuate, perhaps one of the causes of nighttime migraine attacks. Dreaming is the last stage you pass through before waking in the morning; that may be the reason for migraine attacks that greet you at 7 or 8 a.m.

REM seems to be centered in a different area of the brain, the pons, than the other sleep stages. From its location in the pons, we believe that dreaming is one of the most basic of the brain's functions, right alongside heart rate and breathing, which are handled by the same area—and both play roles in migraine. Dreaming's relationship to migraine may also have something to do with the fact that during sleep, muscle control slips away, including those that control the positioning of the tongue, throat, and pharynx, or airway. Even more control is lost during REM. Everyone experiences this to some degree; you can even feel your breathing slowing down and deepening as you drift off. But people with sleep apnea stop breathing altogether, for brief periods of time.

Another source of trouble can be serotonin levels. Evidence points to serotonin as a major player in sleep stages, both dreaming and quiet sleep. And melatonin is involved when there's any change to your circadian, or daily cycle, the pattern of sleep and wakefulness controlled by the release of certain hormones. That is one of the reasons many people connect melatonin to migraine.

I get migraine attacks after I've exercised. Isn't it bad enough I have to work out?

You're getting what's known as *exertion migraine*. It's usually a stabbing pain that doesn't last long. You may be able to avoid this headache if you spend more time stretching before an exercise session. Gradually work up to higher levels of exertion. Follow exercise with a cool-down and some relaxation techniques. Make sure you're drinking plenty of water during exercise; the headache may not be caused by exertion but by dehydration, a common trigger of migraine. Because exertion migraine has symptoms similar to aneurysm and other blood vessel malfunctions, see a doctor to eliminate it as a possible cause. Once you've done that, you know you've found a trigger.

Sometimes it seems as though my ponytail is too tight. Can something that simple be the cause of all the trouble?

Yes, a tight ponytail can be a trigger. This is sometimes called a *hatband headache*, because hats or caps that are too tight can set a headache off as well. A headband has the same effect. Your trigger, then, is pressure on the blood vessels in your scalp.

FIVE

Migraine and Women: The Estrogen Connection

CASE STUDY

Dee was twelve when she first began to get one-sided head-ache with aura. Her mother naturally became alarmed at her child's reports of flashing lights and head pain, and rushed Dee to an ophthalmologist. He implied, none too subtly, that Dee might need psychiatric counseling. A series of doctors and therapists followed. It was years before Dee managed to convince anyone that she had migraine. Even then, her doctor simply recommended that she take a few Advil (ibuprofen) whenever aura began and suggested that the headaches related to lack of sleep. Dee took the Advil and tried sleeping longer, but the pain didn't go away. The attacks just seemed worse on days when she overslept. Moreover, if she was too late with the Advil, she'd get nausea.

Then something happened that sent Dee searching for better answers: She began taking birth control pills and her usual routine of one or two headaches a month suddenly went haywire. Dee began getting migraine attacks on a weekly basis—sometimes two or more attacks in just one week. It seemed obvious to Dee, if not to anyone else, that migraine was related to her periods in some way. She asked around for the names of specialists and came to me looking for confirmation. Dee's history, symptoms, and her own careful observations made the diagnosis a swift one: She had true menstrual migraine. The attacks had begun at puberty, and initially clustered around her period. That regular pattern was thrown into turmoil by the addition of the hormones in her oral contraceptive.

I recommended that Dee use another form of birth control. When she stopped taking the pill, her attacks went back to the old monthly cycle. Dee began a treatment of verapamil, taken just before her period was due. Most of the time now, the two Advil her doctor prescribed really can handle the pain of an attack. If not, Imitrex is her rescue drug. She uses it if her headache is severe and associated with nausea or vomiting. Dee has finally found relief—and vindication. She was right about her migraine attacks all along.

Everyone I know who suffers from migraine is a woman. Do women get migraine more than men? Is migraine a "woman's disease"? The answer to the first question is yes. Women do have more headaches, and are three times more likely to suffer from migraine than men. About 17.6 percent of all women experience at least one migraine attack in their lives, and women who have chronic migraine get attacks more often than their male counterparts.

But that's no reason to label migraine a woman's disease. The answer to the second question is, in fact, a resounding no. There are two and a half million men in the United States alone who suffer from migraine. Migraine is not limited to women alone.

By calling migraine a woman's disease, people are doing all migraineurs a disservice. Male sufferers, already less likely than women to seek help with their health problems, may be further discouraged from seeing a doctor. Or, when they do visit a physician, their symptoms may be misdiagnosed as something else by a doctor who can't shake the belief that only women get migraine. Worse still, labeling disorders in this way reflects a tendency by many to assume that a number of women's health problems stem from psychological factors alone. Like premenstrual syndrome (PMS), migraine was once thought to be an emotional problem—its symptoms were often dismissed as pure hysteria. We now know that both disorders are the result of true physical changes, but that old mindset persists.

Once it is understood that migraine is not a woman's disease, it can still be acknowledged that women are at greater risk for migraine, and that it is important to take a look at the reasons why.

It all comes down to hormones. Hormones are substances produced by your endocrine glands. They control your body's sexual development and your metabolism. The link to migraine in women seems to be centered on two hormones in particular, estrogen and progesterone. Both estrogen and progesterone are manufactured by your body but can be supplemented by outside means such as birth control pills. The same hormones are also produced in men, but in significantly lower levels than in women; therefore, estrogen and progesterone are considered female hormones.

Estrogen regulates the development of some sexual characteristics during puberty, such as the development of breasts, and controls the growth of the lining in the uterus during a woman's menstrual cycle. Estrogen also regulates changes to the breasts during pregnancy and while breast-feeding. Progesterone readies a woman's uterus for the eggs and prevents more eggs from being produced during the months of pregnancy. A woman's body is programmed to release more or fewer hormones at specific times: for example estrogen levels increase radically during puberty. Levels also increase in the first trimester of pregnancy, while a woman is taking birth control pills, and when hormone replacement therapy is being used. These same hormones fall off during the few days before a period, while a woman is breast-feeding, and during menopause.

All of these changes in hormone levels can impact on migraine. The changes are normal but account for many of migraine's odd variations and fluctuations, such as the way attacks can begin at puberty and end at menopause, or the mixed reports about relief from attacks during pregnancy.

Why do hormones have such a strong connection to migraine? No one is sure. But it seems that when estrogen levels shift radically from highs to lows—like they do during the menstrual cycles and menopause—there is some effect on the way serotonin works in the body.

Another factor may be the role prostaglandin plays in migraine. Prostaglandins are substances that are chemically similar to hormones. Among other things, they tell the blood vessels when to open or shut and manipulate some functions of the nervous system. One type of prostaglandin, PGI_2, crops up more often in women who are pregnant, and in patients taking beta-blocker migraine medication, so it seems that headache patients benefit from having more PGI_2. When you learn that estrogen promotes the production of prostaglandin, it becomes clear how fluctuating amounts of the hormone may be involved in migraine pain. It has been shown that women with migraine generally have lower levels of prostaglandins than those without headache. Doctors have also noted changes in the way prostaglandin works in some women who have menstrual migraine. So, in accounting for headache, the levels of prostaglandins may not be as important as the changing ways in which they work on blood cells.

What can we conclude, then, about women and migraine? Simply this: That while migraine is not a woman's disease, it is a disorder that can have an especially profound impact on its female sufferers. While exact links to female hormones remain cloudy, there's much we do know—and many questions about women and migraine that can be answered.

My doctor used the term "true menstrual migraine." What exactly is that?

Headaches are symptoms of menstrual migraine when there is an unmistakable tie to a woman's period. Migraine attacks that appear *only* during menstruation or in the day or two before or after a period—and not at any other time of the month—are called true menstrual migraine. This type of headache tends to be more severe than other types common to women. About 14 percent of all female migraineurs are diagnosed with menstrual migraine, and most of them started getting migraine with their very first period. Many of these women helped their doctors make the diagnosis, because they were already aware of some kind of link to their periods. If you suspect a similar link, plot your headaches and periods on a calendar or in a headache diary. Note when both begin and end. One good thing about this disorder is that you can time your attacks and so prevent them. Unlike other migraine types, where the pain strikes at random during the month, you know exactly when the pain will occur. That means you may be able to prevent the headache from getting a foothold.

I get headaches during my period but also at other times. Does that mean there's no link to hormones?

Menstruation occurs when unfertilized eggs are discharged from the body along with tissues from the uterus. Hormones time this maneuver, and true menstrual migraine happens only during that period and at no other time. However, your hormones are also active during ovulation, when your ovaries are releasing eggs. So, if migraine makes an appearance during your period *and* midway during ovulation, it is called menstrually related migraine. A headache could be linked to your hormones but is not considered either of these types if you get migraine during menstruation or ovulation, but also at other times during the month.

Are one-sided headaches typical of hormone-related migraines? And what are other symptoms?

Yes, hormone-related headaches are usually unilateral. But the side they appear on may switch from one attack to another, or even shift from side to side during an attack. Nausea and vomiting are always associated with this kind of migraine. Some women get symptoms similar to the PMS syndrome: They begin to fill up with fluid, feel lethargic, or just don't feel right; they can't function properly for a day or two. Most women report the typical throbbing pain of migraine; this pain often persists for days rather than hours. Sufferers often can't stand any kind of light or noise and immediately head for their darkened, quiet bedrooms. Children, jobs, any kind of life takes a distant second place to the pain.

What treatments work best on a woman's hormonally related migraine?

It is sometimes difficult to treat menstrual migraine, but some of the newer drugs have been used with great success. With careful use of these medications you can now prevent these painful headaches. Sumatriptan, sold under the brand name Imitrex, has recently been shown to work well in treating this type of headache.

Menstrual migraine also responds to the preventive medication ergotamine tartrate, known under brand names like Cafergot and Wigraine. When taken in the five- to ten-day period surrounding your period, ergotamine may have a significant impact on menstrual headache pain. Menstrual migraine can also be treated with methylergonovine, sold as Methergine; ergonovine, known under the brand name Ergotrate; and injections of DHE-45. Ergomar may also be useful; it is a tablet of ergotamine placed under the tongue and permitted to dissolve without swallowing. Decadron and other cortisone treatments might help, and ketorolac tromethamine has been known to relieve an attack already in progress.

Water pills like Diamox and Moduretic can be used to relieve some of the PMS-like symptoms of menstrual migraine. These pills, called diuretics, can prevent bloating in women prone to water retention, and seem most helpful when taken for a few days before as well as during a woman's period. Like any other medication, take them under a doctor's supervision, since they may have unhealthy side effects.

Nonsteroidal anti-inflammatory drugs, or NSAIDs, may be particularly effective on your moderate or severe headaches if they're taken in adequate amounts prior to your menstrual cycle. Sansert seems effective, too. Cyproheptadine, with the brand name Periactin, is another drug used in treating menstrual migraine or withdrawal headaches that result from stopping the birth control pill. Propanolol and amitriptyline can help as well, if taken just before and while a woman is having her period. Women often augment their migraine medication with something to help their nausea, like Phenergan or Reglan (metoclopramide), because that symptom can be very bad in menstrual migraine.

A treatment option that women can try in an effort to regulate headache pain is to wear an estrogen patch for a few days before their period. The patch releases the hormone in a steady pattern that can ward off headaches. Other women have had luck cutting down on headaches when using estradiol gel, an estrogen supplement applied through the skin. Estrogen use can have side effects, too, so learn all you can from your doctor before you weigh the pros and cons. Before considering either estrogen or a drug as part of your migraine treatment plan, you should read the chapter on drug treatments for more information and consider the alternatives.

What are the nondrug therapies I can use for menstrual-related migraines?

Biofeedback can work wonders for many patients and has none of the negative side effects of estrogen or drugs. Women who have tried everything else for their menstrual migraine attacks, and who have not found relief using medication, have reported success with biofeedback. A good diet can help tremendously, too, since so many food triggers are worse at this time. Increase the complex carbohydrates in your diet, like pasta and rice. Steer clear of known triggers. Exercise seems to improve the situation for women, too, and exertion headaches are less of a danger to menstrual migraineurs. You might notice improvement with a regular exercise regimen around the time of your period. Some women have reported that submerging hands and feet in hot water helped ease the pain. Limited doses of vitamins B_6 and E have been recommended by other migraineurs. Try some of these options and you may find you don't have to take drugs, or need them less frequently.

My daughter just had her first period—and her first migraine. What's in store for her through the next few years?

Many women can date their first migraine to the time they first began menstruating, a point known as menarche. The hormonal changes experienced during puberty may be the first triggers that wake the sleeping gene that carries migraine. A young woman's menarche migraine may last for several weeks and be resistant to any form of medication, even those normally successful in dealing with menstrual migraine. That kind of lingering, incessant pain can be frightening, and a first-time sufferer should definitely be examined by a doctor to rule out other causes for the headache—but if it is migraine the pain will eventually pass. After that first attack, a young woman's headaches will follow a more normal cycle and won't persist for such a long period again. However, your daughter may experience many attacks over the next few years, as she matures and hormone levels ride a roller coaster of peaks and valleys.

My triggers only seem to affect me during my period. Is that unusual?

It isn't unusual for triggers to have more of an impact during menstruation. Many women report that they are extra vulnerable to attack at that time. Stress, in particular, is even more likely to bring on headaches during a woman's period—another reason why migraine is often associated with PMS. Food-related triggers seem to be the most frequent culprits in menstrual migraine, particularly caffeine, chocolate, and alcohol. Alcohol may have more of an effect at this time because the liver has a role in breaking down estrogen and progesterone. Fluctuations in the amounts of these hormones make more work for the liver, which then has trouble performing some of its other diet-related tasks.

My friend gets headaches right before her period. Is it PMS or migraine?

Your friend can answer this question using the same criteria doctors use to determine whether the two are related but not the same disorder: by observing whether her PMS medication works on the headaches and if her migraine medication relieves the range of symptoms of PMS. Studies have shown that no, the treatment for one doesn't do much to relieve the other, and so have determined that the two are separate problems. That's a somewhat simplified explanation, but it is the basis on which doctors often distinguish one disorder from another.

To explain the common timing, some doctors consider migraine to be concomitant to PMS. In other words, it is distinct from that syndrome but occurs at the same time. Why this happens is in some ways still a mystery, but it's clear that hormonal changes are responsible for both. The changes set off a whole host of reactions—some of which cause PMS symptoms, some of which trigger migraine.

The minute I started taking birth control pills, I started getting terrible headaches. Are they migraines?

They might be. Birth control pills have varying amounts of estrogen and progesterone. They fool your body into thinking you're pregnant, so eggs aren't produced or released. When you know there's a connection between changing hormone levels and migraine, it's easy to see that the pill could play a role in your headaches. If you have menstrual migraine, the chances are pretty good that taking the pill will be a trigger for you. Women whose migraine attacks aren't related to menstruation are slightly less likely to be affected.

Birth control pills also have a tendency to destroy vitamin B in your body. This vitamin aids in pain management and dealing with stress. It seems to help in treating migraine. You might consider moderate amounts of a vitamin B supplement if you're taking the pill. Finally, if you find that your migraine attacks started with the use of the pill, or if your headache attacks increase with the use of oral contraceptives, it is advisable to switch to an alternative method of birth control.

If my periods are regular, why do I get attacks?

Even though your periods occur at regular intervals it doesn't mean that estrogen levels in your body are remaining consistent. It's the hormones, not the timing, that are the key factor in menstrual migraine. However, if you're regular or get premonitory signs before your period, you can use that knowledge to treat menstrually related migraine. You may prevent headaches by beginning medication two or three days before your period. In that sense, you're luckier than some migraineurs who take preventive medicine every day during the month to combat their more randomly timed headaches.

Are there any drugs I definitely shouldn't take if I'm on the pill?

There is a rare condition known as migraine-related stroke. It is a matter of controversy whether taking birth control pills can increase your likelihood of having this condition. The pill puts you at greater risk of blood clots that can cause stroke. If the symptoms you usually experience before and after a headache persist after your headache has passed, you may be having a migraine-related stroke. Other signals of this kind of stroke are changes in your migraine's intensity, sensations of weakness or numbness, or new visual problems. In a very few cases, the effects of the stroke are permanent.

Age and smoking also increase the likelihood of migraine-related stroke. Be warned: A woman with this addictive, migraine-triggering habit who is also taking the pill dramatically increases her risk of migraine-related stroke. Therefore, nicotine should be avoided when using oral contraceptives.

I just discovered that I am pregnant. Will my migraine attacks get worse?

On the contrary, between 60 and 75 percent of women experience a decrease in frequency or severity during pregnancy. When a woman is pregnant, her estrogen levels don't fluctuate as much as when she is menstruating. Even though estrogen levels can soar during the last two trimesters, that seems to have less of an effect than the fact that the levels remain *constant* even though they are high. Relief at this time may also occur because women produce more endorphins during pregnancy, especially during the last few months. Endorphins are responsible for the runner's high so many athletes experience and play an important role in the body's management of pain. An unlucky 10 percent of migraineurs have more or harsher attacks while they are pregnant; that's more often the case when their migraine attacks weren't menstrually related in the first place. Some women experience a temporary increase in migraine frequency during the first trimester.

I'm in my second trimester and still getting headaches. Are there any medications that are effective for me and safe for my baby?

Nearly all migraine medications are harmful to a developing fetus, so you should discontinue use as soon as you discover your pregnancy or while you're trying to conceive. Under constant, careful supervision, some women use small dosages of acetaminophen with codeine, hydrocodone, or Demerol while pregnant. Beta-blockers have been used by patients with excruciating pain, although they must be taken in small doses and discontinued about a month before delivery. Because of the possible dangers, an expectant mother should exhaust the possibilities of biofeedback, heat therapy, ice packs, increased rest, and relaxation techniques before turning to drugs. Consult your physician before using any medication (prescription or over-the-counter) during pregnancy.

My sister started getting headaches after she had kids. She never had them before. Is that common?

Recent studies suggest that a small percentage of female migraineurs encountered their first attack while pregnant. Many more experienced their first attack right after delivery. It may be that the abrupt drop in estrogen experienced after giving birth is the trigger that wakes migraine from its sleep. If the onset is during pregnancy, it usually occurs during the first trimester.

I'm breast-feeding. Is medication still a danger to my baby?

In general, women don't want to take medication while nursing a baby, since whatever a mother consumes is also ingested by a breast-feeding child. For some mothers, however, there is little choice—the pain is too great or doesn't respond to any of the nondrug treatments. Risks to infants from most migraine medications are still unclear. Although some studies have been done on animals, very few have tracked the effects of migraine medications on nursing mothers and their children. Still, it's recommended that anyone breast-feeding stay away from ergotamine. Imitrex, the brand name for sumatriptan, has shown up in animal's milk, so it could be another medication to avoid. Other drugs may present a danger as well, so if you're taking medication, be sure to let your doctor and your pediatrician know you are breast-feeding.

What effect will menopause have on my migraines?

The hormone fluctuations that occur naturally during menopause, or are produced by medications taken by menopausal women, seem to be responsible for the 10 percent of women who report a first attack over the age of forty. More often, though, this period in your life is the beginning of the end for migraine.

Menopause, climacteric, or "change of life," as it's sometimes called, is the time when a woman stops menstruating. Most women experience menopause naturally, anywhere from age forty to sixty. That wide age range demonstrates just one of the ways in which menopause is unique from one woman to the next. Menopause symptoms—hot flashes, aches, excess perspiration, irritability, and insomnia—may last anywhere from a few weeks to five years. Symptoms may pass almost unnoticed in some women, or become extremely severe in others. Menopause can also produce osteoporosis, a condition where the bones become thinner and far more brittle. Women can experience early menopause after getting a hysterectomy, if there has been a complete removal of the ovaries.

How does menopause impact on migraine? During menopause, lower levels of estrogen are produced. Once those levels begin to fall, many women experience what seems to be a miraculous relief from migraine.

Could my menopause hormone therapy be responsible for my sudden attack of migraine?

For some, the relief from migraine brought on by menopause is short-lived. Doctors often place menopausal patients on estrogen replacement therapy, or ERT, to deal with conditions like osteoporosis. Because it is manipulating hormone levels, ERT can temporarily worsen migraine in women who have already had attacks or bring them on for the first time in women who have never had one of these agonizing headaches before. ERT can have other negative health effects, so a migraineur should think about alternatives to this therapy or alternative ways of taking the hormones. Taking 2.5 milligrams of progesterone daily with your estrogen therapy may help improve the situation.

Many women reduce the number of headaches they get when they take ERT in patch form. With the patch, estrogen is released in a steady flow, rather than in the peaks and valleys that come from taking it in pill or cream form. This steady level seems to have a very positive effect on headaches.

Before beginning ERT in the first place, though, you should ask your doctor to take a blood test to determine your

existing hormone levels. Don't just assume you need to replace them. If you haven't had a hysterectomy and your estrogen levels are high, you might not need the supplemental
hormone at all, and simply be setting yourself up for migraine. Women with menstrual-related migraine may experience the disappearance of their migraine attacks during
menopause and in later life, while individuals with other migraine triggers continue to have attacks.

So, are hormone replacements a cause or cure for migraine?

During menopause, hormone replacements are more often
a trigger for migraine than a "cure." For some women, they
are the start of migraine woes, bringing on the disorder for
the first time. But for premenopausal women, an estrogen
patch may help. Although it's not a cure, it can be part of a
treatment plan. The patch releases estrogen at steady rates
that can bring migraine relief to nonmenopausal women who
suffer from hormonally linked headaches.

Current scientific evidence suggests that the use of hormone replacement therapy, during menopause and after, may
prevent osteoporosis in susceptible women and reduce the
chance of premature coronary heart disease and Alzheimer's
disease.

Will a hysterectomy help rid me of these headaches?

There is no evidence that hysterectomies help prevent migraine attacks, although many women do report relief after
the operation, just as they do during menopause. However,
there *is* evidence to show that the treatment that follows a
hysterectomy may make migraine worse. Migraine is definitely not an indication of a hysterectomy. After the removal
of their ovaries, women are placed on a therapy that includes
estrogen replacement. This treatment may trigger migraine.
If you're on a program that alternates weeks of estrogen with
weeks of progesterone, you may have more migraine relief
by switching to a daily dose of estrogen alone. Check with
your doctor to see if this is an option for you.

Does that mean periods, birth control, pregnancy, and menopause can all have an impact on a woman's migraine? That's not fair!

Yes, they all play roles in migraine pain. And no, it doesn't seem fair. Luckily, women with migraine have persisted in seeking ways to manage their pain and have found that it is possible to take control of headaches.

SIX

The Young Migraine Sufferer

CASE STUDY
Sam was clutching the engine from his favorite toy train when he first visited me with his mother. The wooden piece clearly gave him a feeling of much-needed security. Sam was barely four years old at the time. He was in my office because the numerous tests he'd been given to discover the source of his stomach problems had all come back negative. There appeared to be no physical reason for the violent vomiting attacks he got so regularly. Many family doctors might have suggested counseling, but Sam's pediatrician knew Sam was a happy, well-adjusted toddler when he wasn't having an attack. That doctor had done his homework and was aware that migraine with young children sometimes takes the form of stomach upset. So, although Sam never complained of headache pain, he was referred to me.

Gentle questioning pried out another clue: Sam's parents noticed a sudden drop in the temperature of Sam's feet and hands just before an attack. Together with the negative test results, this symptom seemed to indicate a case of abdominal migraine—a variety of the disorder that shows up far more often in children than adults.

Before prescribing medication, I suggested that Sam learn biofeedback. Sam was intelligent and playful, so the therapist I recommended made the training into a kind of game. Sam quickly mastered the method of making his hands and feet warmer at the first sign of a chill. The attacks dramatically dropped in number as soon he started using this technique. To Sam, it seemed like a fun magic trick. To manage the attacks that did occur, we placed Sam on a treatment plan of mild medication.

When he got a few years older, Sam's attacks evolved into the more common migraine, and headaches were added to his symptoms. We were able to treat those with the biofeedback as well, and occasional doses of nonsteroidal anti-inflammatory drugs (NSAIDs). As he grows older, Sam's migraine attacks may disappear. If not, the number of options for treating them will continue to grow along with this young sufferer, and he'll be able to find relief as long as he gets migraine.

"Mommy, Daddy, my head hurts!" If that sounds familiar, it's because children complain of headaches more often than any other health problem. Somewhere between 7 and 18 percent of all children get at least one migraine attack. The majority of childhood sufferers are boys—roughly 10 percent fewer girls get migraine until puberty reverses the trend. Some children can expect relief by adolescence, especially boys, but attacks are painfully disrupting to both sufferers and their families while they last.

Once a migraineur learns those numbers and discovers that the disorder may be a genetically inherited trait, their first question is always, "Will my children get it?" Although there's no guarantee that the next generation will suffer from migraine, a migraineur's children are more likely to get headache than those with no family history of the disorder.

Migraineurs can, however, use their own knowledge to make their children's experiences easier. A parent who gets migraine may be more apt to recognize its signs. They can assist doctors in making speedier diagnoses, and are more prepared for taking an active role in treating a suffering child.

So how can a family treat childhood migraine? By learning all they can about this type of headache and exploring the alternatives that work best for children. Knowledge is a powerful weapon, both for you and the child battling the disorder. Be sure children understand that migraine is a sickness, not something they "made happen" because they've been bad.

Many kids convince themselves that headaches are a punishment for some terrible wrongdoing.

Another initial step is simply to take the pain seriously. Believe children when they tell you the pain is like a bomb exploding in their heads or a belt tightening inch by inch. Believe in their aura visions of flashing lights, halos, and dancing figures. That may be easier for migraineurs than for parents who have never experienced migraine's unique symptoms. At the same time, if you get headaches yourself and know first-hand how terrible they can be, you will be tempted to coddle your sick child beyond what is helpful. Protect and soothe your children, but also deal with the situation as matter-of-factly as possible and help your migraineur learn to deal with the pain independently. That can be a delicate balance, but it's one most parents routinely face as children grow.

Because stress is often a trigger in childhood migraine, look for ways to spot and treat it. Exercise is often the best way to address this trigger in young children, so channel their energy toward sports. If competitive sports appear to contribute to stress, look at other options, like bike riding, in-line skating, dance or martial arts classes.

Try not to reward a suffering child too excessively, however much you sympathize with their pain. That can cause rebound headache in much the same way that overmedicating can in adults. The child responds to the gifts or special treatment with feelings of pleasure that the body wants to see repeated. If the only way to get that is by producing headache pain, then your child's body will oblige, however unconsciously. The pain is still real; it's just that the need for attention has become a trigger. To avoid this, praise a child's success in avoiding triggers and using biofeedback or relaxation techniques and treat the actual attack with a more matter-of-fact attitude.

Special treatment for a sick child can lead to other problems as well. It can create another tightrope for parents: balancing concern and attention for a sick child with equal focus on other family members—often on top of your own struggle with migraine. It's not easy. Many parents with sick children suggest frequent family meetings where everyone has a voice in deciding how to handle aspects of the problem that affect the whole group, like family outings cut short or competing bids for attention. You might be surprised at the constructive ideas that follow a few minutes' worth of grousing.

Giving more of the control of managing headache pain into the hands of the child suffering may take pressure off everyone, including the young migraineur. The more hands-on involvement you can responsibly allow children in treating their own pain, the more excited and cooperative they'll be about making behavior changes and exploring the range of headache therapies.

Why do children get migraine?

Children get migraine for the same reason adults get them: it's in their genes. A predisposition to the disorder is passed through a family from one generation to the next. A child's migraine can be triggered by the same things that set off their parent's headaches: stress, something they ate or smelled, or even the strain of a prolonged crying episode.

What other conditions should be considered before arriving at a diagnosis of childhood migraine?

Slightly less than one in twenty children may have a neurological cause for their headaches that isn't migraine, ranging in seriousness from needing a new pair of glasses to having a brain tumor or meningitis. Clearly, the latter two are extremely rare, but doctors must still check every potential source of the headache pain before you arrive at a diagnosis of childhood migraine. The most common causes of headaches are the lowest on the scale of severity, such as problems with a child's eyesight. You may notice that, in addition to complaining of headache, your child is squinting, sitting too close to the TV, or holding books right under his or her nose. You might ask your child if he is having problems reading the board at the front of his classroom. Tooth pain from cavities can also be confused for headache in some cases. A visit to the dentist can eliminate that cause and also temporomandibular joint syndrome (TMJ), which is signaled by grinding teeth and a clicking sound when a child chews. Sinusitis shows up as a runny nose, coughing, pain that gets worse when a child bends over, and postnasal drip. If your child routinely feels pain when the slightest bit hungry or after a meal, ask your pediatrician to check for low blood sugar.

More serious causes should be eliminated, too. If a child gets headache along with a fever, has poor appetite, pain in the stomach and abdomen, and vomiting, have him or her tested for hepatitis. Headache with fever and fatigue could also spell a case of the mumps. Poliomyelitis is polio that's contracted from the oral vaccine or exposure at a location where the disease still prevails. Symptoms are headaches and stomach pains that come back more severely each time, accompanied by a sick, achy feeling not unlike flu. High blood pressure might bring on headaches, nosebleeds, and sudden changes in vision. Meningitis can appear as a follow-up to an ear infection or other upper-respiratory inflammation. Besides head pain, look for vomiting and a stiff neck. Children with meningitis may move very carefully or stay unnaturally still, because tilting the chin downward and doing other maneuvers cause pain. Mononucleosis shows up with rashes, sore throat, fever, swollen glands, puffy-looking eyelids, tiredness, visual problems similar to aura, and pain in the lower stomach along with the headache. Headaches may follow some trauma to the head from a fall or accident. Carbon monoxide poisoning may be the cause of headaches when your child gets them only when being a passenger in a specific vehicle or after spending time in a particular room.

As for brain tumors, keep in mind that only one out of every forty thousand children develops them. Migrainelike symptoms of brain tumor include waking up with head pain, headaches that get worse with each attack, and pain that begins in the neck. But seizures and projectile vomiting are symptoms that tend to show up first.

My child is too young to talk very much. How can I know if she's got migraine, or how can I find out about her pain?

Obviously, childhood migraine is attended by the special difficulties of treating patients who may be too young to tell you where it hurts. However, parents recognize headache pain the same way they sense a child is hungry or needs to be changed: Their baby cries and acts cranky or uncomfortable. Of course, there are other clues, too. If you are a migraineur, you might aid your pediatrician in spotting headache in your child, simply by recognizing the signals you display when having an attack. Your baby may seem more easily irritated than normal. She may squint or turn her head away from even dimmed light sources. She may vomit. Sleep may be disturbed, with no apparent cause for the tossing and turning. Fingers and toes may feel chilly. A child may appear flushed but have no fever, even if she hasn't been active. A small child will frequently rub her head and eyes. Migraine is now suspected to be the culprit when infants repeatedly bang their heads against sides of cribs.

Remember that children are easily distracted and will often ignore the early-warning signs that an older migraineur spots instantly. A very active child may not display any signs at all until the pain becomes intense. So learn to spot subtle changes. Then, try to get your child to describe the pain by equating it to other hurts she has experienced, like a smacked funnybone or bruised knee. Ask her questions that pinpoint the sensation: Was it a stabbing, throbbing, or tugging feeling? Children who have a hard time articulating their sensations should be encouraged to draw pictures of how the pain feels and what their aura looks like. Take these pictures with you when you visit your child's doctor.

What kind of doctor should treat my child's migraine?

Your regular pediatrician can treat childhood migraine. But if attacks arrive almost daily, or don't respond with any of the medications or therapies you've already tried, see a pediatric neurologist or a headache specialist. When you visit your child's doctors, go prepared. Bring notes on your child's particular warning signs, symptoms, the location of the pain, and how long each stage of the attack lasts. Before migraine is diagnosed, doctors may ask you for a detailed family history, including questions about your pregnancy. This will help target testing. Your child may have to undergo some of the same tests as adults, like MRI (magnetic resonance imaging) and CAT (computerized axial tomography) scans.

What type of migraine attacks do school-age children get?

Children's migraine attacks are often very similar to those suffered by adults, although they can be of much shorter duration and sometimes include abdominal distress and vomiting. Some attacks are over in less than fifteen minutes; and most don't last a day. Children can get cluster and tension-type headaches, as well as migraine. Children are also more likely to get some of the migraine variants described in Chapter 2, but those are still fairly rare, even in children.

A typical migraine attack may include symptoms such as aura, numbness of extremities, stomach pains, cramping, nausea, vomiting, diarrhea, slurred speech, vision problems and feelings of confusion or dizziness. Children often get their headaches early in the day; many wake up with them.

Those children who get head pain describe two kinds. The first; the throbbing headache, is usually on one side, accompanied by nausea and other ''sick'' feelings. The second type feels like the brain is being torn or tugged apart. This pain can spread all over the head and may be brought on by tightening muscles.

My eight-year-old suffers from abdominal migraines. What causes this?

This is a form of childhood migraine that differs from adult headache in one very striking way: There is no headache. Vomiting and intense stomachache is abdominal migraine's calling card. Instead of a headache, the child's pain appears as stomach upset and cramping. Children may vomit even on an empty stomach, and the upset may last for hours or days. Vision is blurry, and children feel like they're spinning. They may have quick mood shifts, lose their appetite, or demand specific foods. Young patients may feel very tired or weak and be extremely sensitive to light.

Abdominal migraine shows up cyclically and it's a frequent visitor. This condition is diagnosed largely by eliminating other possibilities. It can strike children when they are very young; some babies as young as one year old have been diagnosed with abdominal migraine.

What do I tell my six-year-old when he asks why he gets headaches?

Tell your child as much as he wants to know—sometimes that may be less than you think. Before reeling out the facts about migraine's basic mechanisms, ask your child why *he* thinks he gets them. Then you can address the specific concerns that spurred the question. He might believe he gets them as a punishment by God for goofing off in school or being mean to a sibling, in which case you can explain that migraine attacks are a sickness like flu, and that they have nothing to do with misbehavior. If a child asks where migraine comes from, you can explain that headaches sometimes get passed along through a family, just like brown hair or big feet. Balance that explanation with some positive trait that has been passed along in your family.

Do children get aura? If so, how do I explain that to a child?

Children do get aura and often have more dramatic visions and sensations than their parents. Children experiencing aura may look dazed, or act like they are hallucinating. They'll accept these symptoms fairly readily once you explain that other people get them as well. In fact, there are even children who find the experience magical, especially once they realize they won't be punished for talking about their visions. What frightens children may not be the aura, but the certainty that adults won't believe their stories of flashing lights and patterns, especially if a child was initially accused of lying about his or her visions. One way to open children up to a discussion about aura is by asking them to draw what they see and feel during that phase.

What can I do for my child besides give her drugs?

Alternatives to drugs should always be explored first in a child's treatment plan. These options can be very effective with children, because they are such experts at learning new things and are open to the idea of increasing conscious control over their bodies. Even children as young as six and seven can learn to manipulate their body's reactions through biofeedback. Children can be trained to recognize their own aura or other premonitory signs and begin biofeedback wherever they happen to be. It can be treated like a game, a race to beat the headache by bringing up body temperature. Like so many other things, kids seem quicker to pick up this skill than their headache-prone parents; they easily master the technique for warming their fingers. Even younger chil-

dren can be taught simple relaxation techniques that include
deep breathing and massaging their hands and feet. You can
also help children by guiding them through behavior
changes, such as staying away from triggers, taking calming
breaths in exciting or stressful situations, sticking to a regular
sleep schedule, and exercising. For children with a light-
sensitive trigger, a strobe light programmed to blink at slow,
regular intervals has been known to help. But the best nondrug medicine seems to be sleep. If a child is too worked up
to sleep, a few minutes of quiet time, a quick set of relaxation
techniques, or some soothing compresses can be very effective in calming the child into sleep. For a more in-depth look
at many of these alternatives, turn to Chapter 9. Treat the
exploration and mastery of these alternatives as an adventure
in order to encourage your child's participation. Emphasize
that controlling the body can be like gaining a magic power.

Isn't aspirin dangerous for babies?

Aspirin contains salicylate, a type of salt. It's the salicylate
that poses the problem, because it can cause inflammation of
the liver and brain, a disorder called Reye's syndrome. The
syndrome's symptoms are similar to those of migraine: headaches, vomiting, and a need for more sleep. Check with your
doctor before giving aspirin to a child under sixteen.

Are any medications safe for children?

Parents often seek other ways to treat their children before
looking toward medication for help. That instinct is a good
one; if you reach for acetaminophen at the first sign of headache pain, your child may not bother learning other ways to
manage the pain. You shouldn't use medication as a child's
first defense against pain, because of drug interactions and
side effects.

If attacks occur more than once a week and don't respond
well to other therapies, however, the benefits of medication
may outweigh the dangers. Be aware, though, that the
smaller the body absorbing the drug, the more extreme the
drug's actions and the body's reactions. Side effects can be
even more apparent in children. In most cases, it is these
effects and other potential problems that make doctors hesitant to use drugs as an initial line of defense for children.

Sometimes, they hesitate because they don't believe your child's pain is "serious" enough to merit medication. Try to find out which concern is behind your pediatrician's choice for your child, and make a decision about the seriousness of the situation together.

Which drugs work best in treating childhood migraine?

Like the medications used for adults, a child's options are divided into abortive and preventive drugs. Most families begin treatment using over-the-counter abortive drugs, which stop a headache already in progress or just beginning. Learn more about the drugs listed here in Chapter 8.

The first drug tried on children is normally acetaminophen, sold under brand names like Tylenol. It is not the most effective drug, but it is the safest, with virtually no side effects. Children often take it with a cola, which helps it work more quickly. Acetaminophen is available in a chewable tablet form for easier swallowing, but there are also liquids and suppositories.

Aspirin-free Excedrin is stronger and has a dose of caffeine built in, but that amount of caffeine can be too strong for children under the age of nine. One of the drug's side effects is sleepiness, which actually may help by pushing your child to seek rest.

Ibuprofen is often the next step; Advil, Motrin, and Nuprin are some of its brand names. This is available in a liquid that goes down fairly easily with young sufferers, but upset stomach and dizziness may result from using this drug.

If the pain is too much for these OTCs to handle, parents can take the leap to stronger drugs like naproxen, available as Aleve, Naprosyn, and Anaprox. It can make your child feel tired and dull. Midrin contains acetaminophen but also a sedative. Its capsule can be emptied into applesauce or drinks, which makes it easy to dose children seven and older. Stomach upset and dulled reactions from the sedative are some side effects of Midrin.

Other drugs used to treat children may include an ergotamine like Cafergot. Butalbital helps your child sleep and comes in several forms: Fiorinal has aspirin, which can be a danger for children; Phrenilin has acetaminophen; Fioricet and Esgic have acetaminophen and caffeine. They are at times extremely helpful in childhood migraine. A dose of one-half of a tablet may be adequate for relief. While on these drugs, children may seem agitated, giddy, or tired, and stomach pain or upset is not uncommon.

If abortive drugs aren't working, the next level tried is preventive medication, which may include any of the following drugs: cyproheptadine hydrochloride (Periactin), an antihistamine used in treating allergies that's taken just before sleep and which also has antiserotonin activity, which may make it more effective than other antihistamines; propranolol (Inderal) and timolol (Blocadren), beta-blockers that should be avoided by asthmatic children; phenobarbital (also its brand name), an anticonvulsant and sedative that treats dazed symptoms; phenytoin (Dilantin), another anticonvulsant. Investigate the side effects these powerful preventives may have on your child.

Other medications may be used to treat problems associated with migraine. Ambien is a drug used to regulate sleep patterns. Amitriptyline (Elavil) and nortriptyline (Pamelor, Aventyl) work on the depression that can trigger or accompany headaches but may also have specific migraine preventing properties.

If a doctor recommends any of the drugs listed here, or another, ask questions! Just because a physician hands you a prescription, doesn't mean you have to accept it without blinking. See what your doctor says about side effects. Ask what other substances interact negatively with the drug. Find out precisely how to administer it and in what dosages. If a doctor is impatient with these questions, explain why it's important for you to know: It's your child.

My child is terrible about shots, finicky about liquids, and hates suppositories. Are there any candy-coated medications?

Ask your pharmacist if the medication you use can be rendered in a flavored lozenge; some of them can. Other pills might be taken with colas which speed the drug action and make a bitter pill easier to swallow.

Are there any triggers specifically common to children?

Children's triggers are pretty much the same as an adult's: changes in light levels, overexertion, dehydration, sleep problems, weather changes, travel, hunger, stress, noise. Particularly common food triggers include some candies, packaged snack cakes, fried foods, hot dogs, bologna, cheeses, chocolate, dairy products, caffeine, and MSG. Asthmatic children may be more sensitive to sulfites they eat in dried fruits, such as raisins, and mashed-potato flakes. A child's consumption of fruit-flavored drinks that use certain dyes such as red #40 and yellow #5 can be a trigger. The caffeine in some sodas may be a trigger, or the trigger could be the insomnia brought on by these late-night sips of caffeine. Children also commonly have pressure triggers like tight headbands or too-snug ponytails.

How can you find a child's triggers?

Start a headache diary with your child. Learn about his or her triggers with queries like the following: Did anything special happen on your bus ride this morning? Did you have any arguments with people in school? What snacks were shared today? Did the headache start right after the movie? Were you especially tired today?

The next step is a modified elimination diet. For a week, serve your children a menu that avoids the food triggers you identified using the headache diary as well as other common food triggers (see page 197). This diet can include allowable vegetables, fresh meats, pasta (without tomato sauce), rice, allowable fruits, and lots of water. Then reintroduce potential triggers, one at a time. Note which sets off a reaction, then remove it from the menu. After a week or two try it again to see if you get the same headache response.

Why does my daughter get migraine attacks whenever she's especially happy or excited?

Excitement of any kind—good or bad—can be a trigger for children because of chemical reactions it sparks in the brain. If you've noticed a relationship between excitement and migraine in your child, work on relaxation techniques together. Be vigilant about situations that could lead to migraine, and be ready to pull your child aside for a few moments of cool-down when emotions run too high. As children get older, they learn to recognize these signs themselves and to control themselves almost unconsciously.

Can too much TV be the culprit behind my son's frequent headaches?

The flickering screens of TV sets and computer monitors seem even more powerful triggers for kids. So, yes, exposure to those changing light patterns can be behind some headaches. Content might be a trigger, too. If your child always gets migraine after an upsetting news report, an excessively violent program, or a show that gets him very excited, switch the channel or encourage relaxation techniques when a likely trigger hits the screen.

My child can't keep anything down when he has a migraine. What should we do about the constant nausea?

Trimethobenzamide (Tigan) and promethazine (Phenergan) can both be helpful in combating nausea. Their side effect of making children feel sleepy is also a benefit, since it encourages rest. Unfortunately, they are administered in rectal suppositories. Although this method is more effective than oral drugs in speeding medication through the body, children often feel that rectal dosing is the final indignity of migraine.

My child's triggers are all foods. How can I help him avoid these triggers?

Helping your child maintain a trigger-free diet can be one of the most basic treatments. But, as any parent knows, persuading kids to eat well isn't always easy. Eat together, and at home, as often as you can. You'll know for sure what your child is consuming, and can guide him to better eating habits by your own example. The best way to steer your child away from trigger foods is to avoid these foods yourself—at least when you're with your child. Children learn many of their habits from mimicking the adults they respect, even unconsciously. You need to be conscious of that instinctive behavior, and use it in your child's treatment. Don't attempt

to force-feed your child. Arguments about food can just rebound. An angry child may deliberately eat trigger foods just
to irritate a parent who has turned the dinner table into a
soapbox.

Instead, from time to time introduce a new, nontrigger
food. Tell your child to try a bite of these new foods, but
don't insist he clean his plate if the reaction is negative. Find
out why your child didn't like it—it was "too mushy," "is
yellow," or "has lumps." Then simply try again some other
night, in a different preparation that masks what he didn't
like the first time.

Downplay the fact that a particular food is good for your
child. Instead, say you want your child to try it because *you*
like it, or because monkeys, bears, or parrots eat it, if that's
the case. Fresh fruits and vegetables are more appealing to
children, and serving them fresh avoids triggers like preservatives and chemicals used in frozen and prepared foods.
Offer raw vegetables, too, which often go over even better
than cooked ones. Involving your child in choosing nontrigger vegetables at the grocery may induce them to eat them.
Plant a garden or windowbox with nontrigger vegetables,
with older children helping in their care. That will make them
more interested in eating the finished product. Older children
will understand the headache-food trade-off.

As soon as they can read, teach children which words to
look for in food labels. Make a game out of it at the grocery
store. Don't shield children from the disorder or the consequences of eating indiscriminately when they're old enough
to understand. They may occasionally make the wrong
choice, but they'll learn from their mistakes and begin to take
control of their own migraine.

Why is lunch such a problem?

Many lunch meats, especially the cheaper ones, can be
potent triggers because of their preservatives. That other
lunchroom staple, peanut butter, is also a known trigger. If
both set off your child's headaches, you'll have to use fresh
meats and find more inventive paper-bag offerings.

How can I protect my child from food triggers when
he's away from home?

If your child is old enough, talk to him about what to
avoid. At the same time, educate the personnel at the places

where your child may eat. Talk with parents of your child's friends about migraine triggers. Provide them with lists of your child's triggers *before* a visit is planned so they'll be prepared in a pinch. Offer to send snacks for everyone when you send your child on a sleepover. Check out the food selections at your child's daycare center or school. Does the staff there understand that this is a disorder with physical causes that can be triggered by certain food chemicals or situations? Can you help them plan a diet for your child, or will they make sure he eats food that you've prepared? Do they have a plan for smoothing over any awkwardness in the lunchroom?

My son is unbearable during his attacks. He's not a baby anymore, though, so what can I do to control his headache-anger?

There are lots of reasons why children with migraine get angry: They are in pain; they're losing out on fun times when they get attacks; siblings may pick on them out of jealousy over all the attention; they may feel like they are "freaks."

There are ways your child can channel that anger, however. Some of them also have the beneficial side effect of lessening headache pain. Offer your child opportunities to learn tai chi, karate, or other martial arts that emphasize concentration. Enroll him in a movement or dance class. Plan family outings that include exercise, such as hikes, canoe trips, and biking. Young children can let out their anger on an inflatable punching bag. Put up a basketball net in the driveway for older kids. Practice relaxation techniques with him. But a very angry child may need counseling to help him deal with his emotions and accept migraine's impersonal nature.

I'm concerned about addiction. Are there any drugs that hold this special danger for my teenager?

The same drugs that pose addiction and rebound problems for an adult can affect an adolescent. Teenagers are especially at risk for rebound headache from addiction to nonprescription drugs they can purchase themselves. If your teenager reacts negatively to lectures from you, ask his or her doctor to explain the risks.

How can I make my teenage daughter more responsible about her treatment plan?

Teenagers are in a constant struggle with their parents for control, and migraine can become a battleground. Try to find less confrontational ways to encourage treatment. Provide information in a low-key way, so your teenager can use her own intelligence to make decisions. If she's like most teenagers, she's not going to let you make those choices for her. Point out celebrities and sports stars she might respect, like the basketball great Kareem Abdul-Jabbar, who have learned to manage their migraine attacks or other disorders. Subscribe to women's and fitness magazines that emphasize health issues. Explore opportunities for your teenager to volunteer at a local hospital. Seeing the results of poor health management may make those consequences clearer than a dozen lectures. If you have a child who likes to be a leader, let her know about the networks of support groups. Perhaps she'd like to start one for other teenagers in the area. Plug her in to the Internet; some teenagers are happier discussing their disorder with faceless sufferers. Give your children a voice in choosing their own doctors. Encourage sports that focus on control of the body *and* mind, such as tai chi, karate, and dance. Let teenagers try treatments you may not be tempted to use, such as acupuncture, chiropractic alignments, and massage. Help if you can, with the cost of membership to a gym that attracts lots of young people.

Counseling is an option for teenagers with the disorder, since they become less apt to listen to their parents' suggestions about treating migraine and since some stress-triggers may originate at home. Obviously, other sources of stress may be ones that teenagers are reluctant to discuss openly with parents for fear of judgment, such as sexual tensions and peer pressures. These could be addressed by a professional therapist in a counseling situation.

The use of biofeedback can be particularly effective in teenagers. And it can be introduced with several novel techniques that permit control by the teenager and which use instrumentation which is nonthreatening. In fact, some of the computer tools that we use can be fascinating for an intelligent youth. The parent may want to connect with a local headache center that is conducting studies with adolescents and migraine. My personal experience has been that teen-agers are extremely cooperative and compliant with treatment when the physician and nurses are very careful about explaining their disorder and the drugs that will be used. This age group is often the most rewarding to work with.

Are any drugs particularly dangerous to teens?

Beware of a combination that could cause serious side effects. The antibiotic tetracycline and vitamin A are both acne treatments that, when used together by a migraine-prone teenager can cause a buildup of spinal fluid that puts pressure on the brain.

How can I explain my child's many migraine-related absences to school officials?

First, you should work with your child to cut down on absences as much as possible. Develop strategies a child can use in school, such as biofeedback and relaxation techniques. Talk to school personnel about providing a place for your child to lie down until an attack is over. It's better for him to excuse himself for a half hour than to head home and miss the rest of the school day. Educate school workers on the seriousness of this problem.

Remember, though, that even the most understanding school principal has to abide by state rules governing the number of absences allowed. If your child is experiencing a period of increased attacks, you may need to explore home schooling options until you find a treatment plan that puts your youngster back on track. When your child goes back to school, let teachers know if your child is on drugs that can alter moods or have other side effects that impact school performance. Work with them to find ways to deal with the problems that this might bring.

How should I prepare the school nurse?

Meet with the nurse to make sure he or she knows about migraine and about your child's unique attacks. Give the nurse a list of your child's medications, and keep the list updated. Introduce your child to the nurse at that meeting, too. You don't want their first encounter to occur when your child is screaming in pain. Also, keep track of personnel changes and repeat this procedure if there is a new nurse.

My child only gets migraine attacks at school. What's the connection?

Stressful situations in school may be a trigger. However, the real culprit behind getting migraine attacks in school may be a phobia about getting migraine attacks at school. This stress usually follows that first school attack, when your child may cry or vomit in front of classmates. Few things seem more humiliating. Fear of being labeled with cruel tags by classmates can make children anxious about returning to school. That fear causes a vicious cycle of pain: An attack occurs randomly at school, the child becomes anxious about getting another attack, the stress then triggers more migraine attacks.

How can you calm a child's fears about attacks at school? Take time to talk about it. Agree that having migraine attacks away from home can be frightening, but remind your child that lots of good things happen at school that balance it. Guide your child into talking about those good things. Plot a course of action together: What should your child do when he feels an attack coming on? Who will help him at school? Practice ways he can control migraine there. Encourage your child to believe that he has some control over the disorder, even when away from home.

Can stress possibly be a factor in my seven-year-old daughter's migraines?

A child of any age, even an infant, can feel anxiety and tension. Pay attention to how your child acts when under stresses you know about, such as performance or a test. Is she cranky, quiet, or clingy? Is she easily irritated, tired, or fearful? If that same behavior shows up at other times, or in levels beyond what's normal for that child, a stress you're not aware of might be the cause.

Children are often more sensitive to their surroundings than parents believe. They can sense tensions and react with stress symptoms. So ask questions: Did something make you mad? Did anyone hurt your feelings? Do you feel safe? What happened at school? Listen closely and you may hear answers repeated after each attack, displaying a clear pattern. Once you've spotted your child's stress triggers, gently point them out to your child, along with suggestions for ways of dealing with them. ''See how when you get all excited and mad about losing a game, you can get a headache? Do you think that taking some deep breaths and thinking about your cat might help?''

Rest and relaxation are the best ways for children to deal with stress. If your child's schedule is full of planned activities, cut back. Even if your child enjoys them, too much of a good thing may be just too much. Imaginative play can also help release tension. Exercise starts chemical reactions that reduce stress, too. If the stressful situation can't be resolved, get counseling for your child. It can provide the necessary relief for situations that trigger the migraine and suggest other methods a child can use to defuse stress.

My poor child is so depressed from pain and debilitation. What can we do to help her deal with migraine's emotional toll?

Be supportive and encouraging. Work on helping her take control of the migraine. On the other hand, if your child's headaches are chronic and debilitating, don't allow her to feel ''weak'' for giving in to the pain. Actively search for treatment options together, and in the meantime connect your child with support groups of fellow sufferers. Find out if there are other kids in your town with migraine, and start your own support group, modeling it like a playgroup for younger children. A child often feels the whole family suffers because of her. Guilt can be a terrible burden for a migraineur of any age. So work with other family members to find ways to deal with the disorder. Let your child know her family and friends are a unified team that will work together to make this pain manageable. Show your child she is not alone with migraine pain.

SEVEN

The Treatment Approach

CASE STUDY

"This can't be migraine. A headache can't be causing all this." That's what Dana said before I made a diagnosis of migraine in her case. Several doctors had already formed other opinions about what was causing Dana's problems. They thought she was a schizophrenic or was delusional. She was imagining the pain, they insisted, and most certainly hallucinating her visions. Dana routinely saw strange figures jumping around and dancing lights. Geometric patterns would shoot by. Sometimes a gaping black hole would be punched out of her field of vision. She heard sounds that weren't there. Then the pain would strike, like a *"flashing screw"* that seemed to bore into her head. Loud noises during an attack made her whimper; bright light made her cry. When the pain was gone, Dana couldn't move from her bed for at least a day. But when she got up the next morning, she would be almost giddy with happiness.

Her doctors weren't the only ones who thought she was crazy—Dana was almost convinced of it, too. But she wanted to be sure. She insisted on being referred to a neurologist, who then sent her to me. I took her history and asked about other family members who had headaches. I listened to a list of symptoms that had gone almost unnoticed in the chaos, such as cold hands and feelings of nausea. Dana showed me drawings of her visions. Then we talked about migraine. At first skeptical, Dana then lit up when she learned about aura.

111

*We traced her first attack, dating it soon after she began
taking birth control pills. We designed a chart to monitor
her attacks and found them clustered around her periods.
That had led some to dismiss her attacks as symptoms of
PMS—or worse, hysteria—but Dana was beginning to know
better. The signs were all there, all pointing to migraine.*

*Once she began treatment for migraine, with biofeedback,
ergotamine, calcium blockers, and a watchful diet, Dana got
dramatic results. She was never crazy. Luckily, she was persistent. Dana had just needed to find the right treatment—
for the correct disorder.*

"*I should be able to deal with this myself. After all, it's
just a headache, right?*"

"*I've been to six doctors already and nobody's been able
to do anything to help.*"

"*A headache specialist! Who can afford that?*"

Two out of every three people who have migraine aren't
currently seeing a doctor about their migraine attacks. That
may not seem like such a startling statistic at first, but when
you consider the staggering number of people who get migraine attacks, it becomes clear that many millions of people
out there are suffering needlessly. Needlessly? Yes! Approximately 90 percent of patients who seek help in developing
a treatment plan get some kind of relief. That's a truly phe-
nomenal success rate.

So why don't people rush to get medical help the minute
migraine rears its ugly head? There are many reasons, most
of them what we call migraine myths. It's only when people
discover the truth behind the myth that they realize the benefits of seeking help.

Because of its genetic connection, migraineurs generally
come from a long line of migraine sufferers. There may be
a family tradition of stoically accepting the pain. "Just lie
down until it's over—there's nothing you can do about it"
may be the philosophy a migraineur grew up with. The reality is, there's plenty you can do about it, and you need help
finding out just what that is.

Some people feel embarrassment or guilt over admitting
they need help with their headaches. They've been pro-

grammed by people who have dismissed their pain into thinking they don't have anything to complain about. "It's only a headache" is the all-too-frequent phrase that greets migraineurs. Too many times it's coming from the first doctor a migraineur does consult—which discourages them from ever seeking help again. As we know, though, it's not just a headache. A migraineur should feel no more shame over seeking treatment than when consulting a doctor about a broken leg, diabetes, or a heart problem.

Another barrier to treatment is fear that physicians will "find something really serious" and will say there's nothing that can be done. Many people think it's better to live with the pain and uncertainty than to have their worst fears realized. The odds are very slim, less than 15 percent, that your headache indicates a disease more serious than migraine. But that 15 percent is reason enough for anyone with chronic or severe headache to get help at least once. For instance, if twenty thousand people read this book, one or two of them might be suffering from severe hypertension rather than migraine. When migraine *is* found to be the primary cause, it may not be a question of life and death, but quality of life that can be improved with help from some experts.

Cost factors often play a part in a person's decision not to get medical help. It has been shown that migraine more often strikes those with low incomes, families that are the least likely to have the finances for expert medical treatment. Even when enrolled in a medical plan, patients rely on doctor referrals for specialized care. If a physician is unwilling to make a referral, a sufferer may feel trapped and stop pursuing help. Patients might not be aware that there are low-cost options for their treatment. If they're in a plan, they may not know that they can switch doctors until they find one who will work with them, that second opinions are often covered, and that they may appeal their plan's decisions about the reimbursement of medical costs.

Finally, a migraineur may be under the impression that the only medications available are those purchased over-the-counter (OTC). Certainly the ads on TV persuade you to believe that's the best way to treat your headache. When those drugs don't work, migraineurs simply give up on finding ways to combat the pain. In truth, OTC drugs are only

a tiny fraction of the options available for battling migraine—
and more treatments are being discovered each year. Not all
of these treatments are drugs. A specialist can help you discover new ways to relieve your pain.

So, if any of those reasons were preventing you from seeking help, toss them out the window. The reasons to seek help
are far more compelling: Your headaches could be less frequent, less painful, and vanish more quickly. Treatment can
also help you find ways of dealing with the stress of headache, and it can let others understand migraine's effects on
you. Only 6 to 15 percent of patients who work with doctors
don't get relief. Some of those sabotage themselves by re-
fusing to take control of their own treatment. Are you ready
to get help—and help yourself? As you explore your treatment options, don't settle for less than cutting your headache
pain in half.

How do I know it's time to see a doctor?
"Don't try this at home!" That warning is all too true in
diagnosing migraine. Self-diagnosis is both difficult and dangerous in any disorder with head pain as a symptom. Just
because you've always had headaches doesn't mean you
should make your own diagnosis of migraine or avoid seeking help. Remember that approximately three hundred other
conditions have headache as a symptom. Complacency on
the part of patients is only acceptable if they've been diagnosed by a doctor and know for sure they're not harboring
some other illness. Once a diagnosis is made, you can begin
taking over the management of your headaches. What signs
of migraine should spur that first diagnostic visit? See a doctor to get a diagnosis of migraine if your headaches fall into
one of these categories.

- You get headaches on a regular basis, once a month
  or more frequently.
- Your headaches are disabling enough to keep you
  home from work or school.
- Your headaches last for hours or days.
- The pain doesn't respond well to OTC pills or, if
  these drugs do work, it's only when you take more
  than the suggested dose.

- You have vomiting and nausea along with your headache pain.
- You have vision problems and other disturbances relating to your senses.
- You experienced your first attack over the age of forty-five. Migraine may not be the primary disorder in that case. In patients this age, persistent headaches may be a symptom of an inflammatory disease of the arteries in the head, a serious condition that can cause blindness in a matter of days. Or glaucoma could be a culprit. Glaucoma is not related to migraine, and migraineurs get it no more often than others, but it appears with more frequency in people over forty-five. At this age, headaches might signal a serious lung problem rather than migraine.

If you've been diagnosed with migraine but haven't seen a doctor in some time, and you experience one of the following, it's time for another appointment.

- Attacks are gradually getting worse and worse, lasting longer and longer or coming more frequently.
- A headache attack doesn't follow your usual pattern; there's some kind of change.
- You get an exertion headache that comes on with exercise, a difficult bowel movement, coughing, or sneezing.
- A headache arrives from out of the blue, with no warning signals or aura.
- Your vision, speech, or balance is affected, or other neurological symptoms suddenly appear.
- An attack lasts longer than thirty-six hours.
- You get headaches following a blow to the head.

What kind of doctor should I approach first?

Begin your treatment with what health plans call your primary care physician, also known as an internist or general practitioner. Your history may warrant a migraine diagnosis almost right away. If migraine is difficult to diagnose, your primary physician may refer you to medical specialists.

These might include opthalmologists, dentists, orthopedists, endocrinologists, allergists, or gynecologists. If you seem to be spending a lot of time and money being shuffled between many specialists who seem mystified, ask for a referral to a neurologist or headache specialist. Trips to neurologists can eliminate very serious brain-related diseases and can establish a diagnosis of migraine, but may not offer the best treatment. Neurologists may be less interested in migraine than in the other disorders they treat. A headache specialist or headache clinic is your best bet for developing a treatment plan for chronic headache.

If you choose to make the shift from primary care physician to a headache specialist, you aren't insulting your doctor. Primary care physicians are aware of how thinly they must spread their expertise, and they respect the need to look for more specialized help elsewhere. Acknowledge that you've worked well together, but that it's time to add more players to the team.

When should I go to the emergency room?

Many of the migraineurs in emergency rooms are those who aren't seeing a doctor for help and are desperate for medication to take away the pain. But even patients under a doctor's care should be alert to new symptoms that send up a red flag. These may indicate a new condition, so seek immediate care. If an attack is more agonizing than any headache you've had before, get help right away. If you're getting neurological symptoms you don't normally have, such as vision problems, slurred speech, a dazed or dizzy feeling, memory loss, or limbs that feel weak, numb, or paralyzed, it's a sign that something else might be wrong. Fever or a stiff neck along with a headache may signal meningitis and should be checked promptly.

If you think something is wrong and emergency room personnel seem to dismiss you once they hear a history of migraine, insist on seeing a doctor. It's not necessary for these people to like you—it is necessary that you be checked for conditions that mimic migraine and are far more dangerous.

How can I find a good doctor?

"Can I squeeze in a quick trip during lunch?" Many people choose their doctors by location, putting the most emphasis on a nearby address. That's probably how you should choose a laundry service or pizza shop, but is it really any way to choose a doctor? Use the same care and concern in choosing a physician that you would when making any kind of major investment, such as selecting a house or choosing a college. You're making an investment in your health that has implications just as far-reaching. When searching for good doctors, look at their flexibility, patience, understanding, honesty, and breadth of knowledge—not mileage from your home. Of course, except for knowledge, it's hard to assess these qualities from entries in managed-care handbooks or the directories found in your local library. So, while you should certainly check out a doctor's credentials and affiliations, it's important to find other sources of information that might tell you even more.

Ask your primary care physician or other doctors to recommend someone. Who would *they* call if a loved one suffered from migraine? The nearest teaching hospital can recommend physicians; call the office and talk to staff. Headache associations such as National Headache Foundation (NHF) and the American Association for the Study of Headache (AASH), listed in the chapter on resources, may be able to direct you to a reputable doctor or clinic. The NHF has regional support groups for headache sufferers. Call them and inquire if one exists in your locale. If you contact the NHF, they will refer you to a local practicing physician member. Look for local magazine articles naming the "best-of" doctors in your area or biographical sketches. Ask your librarian to help you find migraine-related works written by nearby doctors. You may want to call the physician's office and ask if the doctor has written any articles on migraine attacks and how you could get hold of them to discover whether you respect their treatment philosophies and approaches.

Once you've got a name, drop by to look at the office. Don't be afraid to ask questions about the doctor. If the doctor's office is reluctant to answer them, that's an answer in itself. Find out how many of the doctor's patients are being treated for migraine and other headache complaints. However competent that doctor may be, only one with a high percentage of migraine patients is likely to keep up to date on the disorder or have a wide range of experience to apply to your treatment. Schedule an appointment as soon as possible—don't wait until you're in the middle of an attack to meet. Don't feel that you're being too finicky if you speak with several doctors in your search for the right one. Another suggestion is to contact your local or regional hospital and inquire whether any headache research studies are conducted there or whether they can refer you to a physician involved in headache research.

What if I don't like my doctor after a few visits?

Finding the right doctor is very important, particularly in migraine. After all, you're both in this for the long haul. The odds are that you'll find a treatment, but that it won't happen overnight. So you and your doctor should be forging a partnership that will last. If a rapport is not happening, it may be time to get a new referral. That may not necessarily mean that your doctor was a poor choice; even the best specialist may not be a perfect fit with a particular patient. If, however, you've worked your way through a dozen specialists, you should take a look at your own role in these partnerships and examine why they aren't working.

What questions is my doctor likely to ask me?

For many disorders, taking a patient's history is important; for migraine, it is essential. Because there is no test for migraine, the only way for doctors to make a diagnosis is by taking a patient's history and eliminating other potential causes of headache for which tests exist. It's basically a process of elimination. What is a history? It's an in-depth interview about your past migraine attacks, lifestyle, environment, and emotional state—in short, it's a pretty complete biography. Be prepared for a lot of questions. Here are some your doctor may ask you: How old were you when you got your first headache? Do you recall any special circumstances that seemed to trigger that first headache? What triggers bring on headaches now? What is your headache pain like—is it throbbing, stabbing, tugging, squeezing, dull, or sharp? How often do you get headaches? Do you have aura? What is your aura like? Where is the pain in your head? Does it move from its original location during an attack?

How quickly does the pain come on? Does the headache go away for a time, or is it constant? What time of day do you usually get migraine? What are your other symptoms before, during, and after an attack of headache pain? What happens after the pain goes away? Has your headache recently changed? Do you get more headaches now than in the past? Does the pain seem to be getting worse? What makes your headache worse during an attack? What seems to help alleviate the pain? What kinds of tests have you had, and what were the results? Have you tried relaxation or other techniques for reducing pain? Are all your headaches the same? What is your sleeping pattern like? Have you lost or gained weight recently? Are you taking any drugs or medications? Have you had any surgery in the past? Do you ever have a fever during an attack? Can you recall any childhood illnesses or allergies? Have you ever experienced a blow to the head? Be prepared with a medical history. If you can't recall childhood diseases, or even if you had headaches when young, ask relatives what they recall or look through old records.

There's one more question you'll get at some point: How will you be paying for this? That shouldn't be the first question you hear in a doctor's office, but it's one you should expect.

What questions should I ask my doctor?

You'll have plenty of questions specific to your treatment as you progress. Don't be afraid to ask any of them, no matter how basic they may seem. A first visit, though, will cover broader ground. You might ask a new doctor to explain the causes of migraine, to see if he or she is current on the biochemical theories now being studied.

Other questions could include: How interested are you in migraine? How do you keep up to date? How many headache patients do you have, and how many have gotten relief? What level of relief can I expect? What is your goal with my headache? What do you see as our plan? What can I do to help myself? Can I get a treatment plan in writing? What happens when a particular strategy doesn't work? How do you feel about nondrug therapies? How do you treat chronic pain? Do you work with other specialists? How long does treatment usually continue? How much time is spent on a visit? How can I get answers to questions between appointments? For the vast majority of people, cost is a consideration and a real concern when seeing a doctor, so some of your questions will be financial ones: What are my payment options? What happens if I can't afford to continue treatment? How expensive are the drugs and other alternatives we'll be exploring? How can your office help me deal with any insurance problems that come up?

Other questions will cover practical issues that may help you plan future appointments: How long should I expect to wait when I have an appointment? How many patients are booked for the same time slot? Can I phone to see if you're on schedule?

What kinds of tests do doctors give to diagnose migraine or to rule out other disorders?

There are many tests that can be involved in arriving at a diagnosis of migraine. You can eliminate the need for some simply by providing your doctor with your previous records, especially any x-rays or scans. Be sure to pass along the films, rather than a lab's interpretation. Your specialist might be able to spot something missed during those previous reviews. Contact the office of your primary care physician or previous specialist to arrange for transfer of those records.

During a first appointment, expect a standard physical examination, followed by a neurological checkup that tests your reactions to an assortment of stimuli. You may be asked for blood and urine samples for laboratory work. If the results of these tests are normal, if your history reveals a long chain of migraineurs in your family, if you display a host of classic migraine symptoms and no other symptoms are present, a diagnosis of migraine may be reached without going any further. If, however, you're foggy on your family history or have a background of other conditions that mimic migraine, more tests are the only way to eliminate masqueraders.

Before having a test done, ask what it is, how it's administered, why you need it, and what effect it might have. Each test prescribed for you should be fully explained to you in advance. There are only one or two exceptions to this—reflex and reaction tests, where knowing what's coming up would defeat the purpose of the exam. In every other case, though, you should know in advance exactly what will happen and why. An electroencephalogram (EEG) is occasionally ordered and is a noninvasive study. It has limited value but can be of diagnostic help to the neurological or headache specialist.

I've been told I need neuroimaging. What is that?

Neuroimaging is a system that allows doctors to map cross-sections of your body, one layer at a time. A scan of your brain, for instance, would show one thin ''slice'' after another, working from the top of your head down to your neck. One method of neuroimaging is done with computerized axial tomography, commonly called a CAT or CT scan. You may need an injection of a contrast agent, a harmless chemical that will make certain elements show up better in the scan. CAT scans are particularly accurate in showing what's happening in the sinus area or in detecting strokes and hemorrhages.

Magnetic resonance imaging, or MRI, is another type of scan. It's used to see if there's anything wrong with your body's basic structures and is sensitive enough to show reduced blood flow through your brain's tiny arteries. MRI uses powerful magnets that affect your body on a cellular level. These scans are less invasive and are more sensitive than other methods of checking for tumors and blockages, such as angiography. They may be more successful than other tests in spotting things like head trauma or TMJ (temporomandibular joint syndrome). MRI scanners are being found in more and more clinics and hospitals today. The original scanner was a long, sealed tube that made many patients feel uncomfortable, even trapped. Some locations now have equipment that isn't so claustrophobic, although some sensitivity is lost. If you're prone to claustrophobia and open MRI scanners aren't available, see if a sedative can be administered to help you through the process.

Neuroimaging scans are expensive but can be essential tests in cases where history doesn't point to a diagnosis of migraine. Other scans may include magnetic resonance arteriography (MRA) or magnetic resonance spectography. Skull x-rays may be done in place of these scans, since they are less expensive, although they're less sensitive, too, and in fact may be of very little value in the diagnosis of headache disorders.

What is a PET scan?

Positron emission tomography, or PET, is a very sophisticated scanning technique that uses isotopes to find out what's going on inside your head. The isotopes are harmless radioactive chemicals injected into your system. Positrons are released as these isotopes decay. They cluster in areas of greater brain activity, and those areas are then recorded by the scanner. PET scans made during attacks have been used to support arguments that there is a biochemical cause behind migraine.

What is a lumbar puncture?

This test is more commonly known as a spinal tap. A lumbar puncture is sometimes performed when it seems that hemorrhaging from a brain tumor or an aneurysm may be the cause behind a sudden onset of headaches. A spinal tap can also detect some infections. A doctor first measures your cerebrospinal fluid pressure, to be sure that removing some will not cause problems. Fluid is then withdrawn, and the sample is tested.

When done properly, the spinal tap produces only mild discomfort, but some people have had more painful experiences. The value of spinal taps in migraine testing is debated, but some doctors use them. Be cautious, though, if a doctor recommends this test right off the bat, unless there are signposts pointing to another condition affecting your nervous system.

Is it true that thermography can confirm a migraine diagnosis?

Thermography is a test that charts your body's various temperature "zones"—in other words, it gives you a picture of the hot and cold spots in your body. Some people believe that you can predict the risk of disorders by looking for areas that are either hotter or colder than normal. It is true that many migraineurs display a cold patch during this test. However, this test's value in reaching a diagnosis of migraine is not widely accepted. Ask why your doctor considers it necessary if this test is recommended.

On my first visit, the doctor asked me all sorts of questions about my family and social life. Is this some kind of psychological test?

Your doctor may ask you questions that appear to be a sneak psychological evaluation or intelligence test. These could include a review of historically significant dates, a description of what you had for lunch yesterday, a step-by-step description on how to tie a shoe, an explanation of what was meant by a famous quote, or questions about how you're getting along with your family that week. Your doctor should explain that these questions are designed to show if damage has occurred in certain areas of the brain known to process this kind of information. Some inquiries are engineered to sniff out potential stress triggers. If your doctor doesn't ask you questions like these, an important part of your treatment program is being ignored.

I've been to several neurologists and other physicians. What can some other specialist do for me?

The more narrowly you focus on something, the clearer certain details become. The same is true with health issues. Internists attempt to keep up to date on medical advances concerning all aspects of the body—a truly monumental task. A neurologist has a slightly narrower focus but still covers a lot of ground. A headache specialist concentrates on a single complaint and can therefore focus all energies on the treatment of that kind of pain. Specialists are more likely to see the latest test results, learn about new medications or alternatives, and observe the gamut of symptoms displayed by the disorder—and be able to apply that experience to your migraine.

I'm enrolled in an HMO. Can I trust their doctor referrals?

Don't assume that a health maintenance organization's referral is going to be inadequate. More and more respected specialists are adding their names to those rosters. Just follow the suggestions given above for finding a good doctor. Ask your HMO plan for the credentials and affiliations of potential doctors. Find out how many migraine patients they treat. Interview the doctor. If you're not satisfied, ask for another referral. Keep at it until you find a doctor you do trust, because this partnership may last quite some time. Allow a couple of visits to see if the chemistry or your opinion improves. These visits are usually covered in full if the specialist is an in-network doctor.

Will a female doctor be more sympathetic and understanding of my hormone-related migraines?

Any good doctor should be able to treat a woman with hormone-related migraine attacks. And a poorly informed female doctor might be just as unsympathetic as an uninformed male doctor. If you feel that your care is being dismissed, that you're being labeled as "hysterical," then by all means look for another doctor—of either sex. But if the problem is a feeling of discomfort when discussing your health issues with a male doctor, and you're otherwise satisfied with your care, try to work through it by talking with your doctor. When you present your concern to him, his matter-of-fact manner may put your discomfort to rest. If, however, you find yourself unable to discuss crucial details with a male doctor, then certainly seek out a female specialist. The level of care may not change, but if your confidence level improves, then the switch will be worthwhile.

What do I do if my doctor thinks I'm exaggerating the pain (I'm not), or doesn't believe my pain is real?

If you're dissatisfied with the way a doctor is handling your care, speak up. Talk about your concerns, and invite your doctor to explain the actions that prompted your suspicions. If you aren't satisfied with the response, switch doctors. First, be sure that a lack of belief in your pain is really what's behind your doctor's behavior. If your physician conducts what seem to be psychological tests, it may simply be part of a neurological exam to reveal damage to areas of the brain. Or doctors may be probing to find triggers that relate to stress. Did your doctor recommend that you see a psychiatrist? That doesn't necessarily mean your pain isn't taken seriously, only that your doctor is recognizing the psychological side to headache pain. Counseling can help you manage one of migraine's primary triggers, stress, and help you deal with the frustration brought on by chronic pain.

Listen to how your doctor questions you about the levels of pain you experience during your attacks. If your doctor took a thorough medical history, performed an exam, obtained samples for lab tests, has supported referrals to other specialists, works closely with you to define your pain and rate it, and uses your ratings to guide treatment, then your pain is probably being taken seriously. If, however, your doctor appears uninterested in rating your pain, prescribes an antidepressive drug as the first line of defense instead of an abortive medication that treats the biochemical sources of migraine, and is reluctant to discuss future plans for treating your pain, then you should look for help elsewhere.

My doctor and I have been searching for an effective treatment for almost a year with no luck. Does that mean my doctor's no good?

Fighting migraine is highly individual. It's true that some patients find relief with the first drug or alternative treatment they try. Most, though, need a lot more time to find the right combination of elements that will work on their headaches. Does your physician keep current on new treatment options? Does your doctor respond with more suggestions when you report failure of a certain treatment? Have you been working with treatments that target the sources of headache pain, such as blood vessel flow or changes in your levels of serotonin or estrogen? If yes, then you may simply need to experiment some more. But first, express your concerns. If you're discouraged, share that with your doctor. On the other hand, if you feel your treatment isn't focused, that your doctor isn't working with you to find new treatments, or that your physician is simply uninformed about alternatives, you may want to find a new doctor or ask for a referral to a specialist.

What should I do if my doctor seems too cautious about trying new strategies?

First, be sure you're allowing enough time for existing strategies to work and aren't simply looking for a short cut where none may exist. If you want to continue working with your present doctor, ask about other options and see if he or she is committed to learning more about these alternatives. Find out whether your doctor's caution stems from concern over your particular history and medical background; perhaps some medications aren't safe for you to use. If you're seeing a specialist and have doubts about your care, it's your right to ask for a second opinion. It's no reflection on a physician's skill to request another viewpoint.

How can I communicate my concerns about how we're treating my migraine without sounding like I'm arguing with or doubting my doctor?

You're allowed to have questions about your health. Don't let fears about being labeled a difficult patient get in the way of receiving the treatment that's best for you. However, remember that you get results that better serve your needs if you discuss problems with someone in a nonconfrontational way. Explain that you're worried, and use language that will begin a discussion, not start an argument: "I'm concerned about this; can you explain what I can expect?" or "I'm not sure why this happened; will you go over it with me again?"

I have trouble understanding my doctor when we talk about the causes of my migraine. How can I get doctors to use plain English?

The problem is that doctors think they *are* speaking plain English; the terms and technology are so familiar to them, it's easy for them to forget that patients don't share the same background. But why should a patient know what beta-blocker or scotoma means? Some migraineurs are afraid of seeming "dumb," though, so they don't ask for explanations. Consequently, a lot of information gets lost in the shuffle. Don't hesitate to stop a discussion and ask for something to be clarified. If you're still feeling lost, suggest that your doctor explain it in language a child could understand. That's not a reflection on your understanding; it's just a trick to make doctors think about the vocabulary they're using. Take notes during your doctor's instructions; in the stress of the moment it's easy for things to go in one ear and out the other. Before leaving a doctor's office, ask what time of the day is good for calling with questions. Then actually make the call if you're not clear on something. Finally, you might try familiarizing yourself with the vocabulary of migraine *before* your appointment. Use the glossary of this book as a guide.

My doctor just gives me a prescription and sends me home. How active should I be in my own treatment?

You have a right and a responsibility to become involved in your own care. Think of you and your doctor as a team, equal partners in fighting migraine. Your doctor brings expertise to the table, but so do you. You know your own pain better than anyone. And while your doctor may be a source for medication and other ideas for treatment, only you can implement them and make them work. The exchange of information and issues should flow both ways. Take notes at home about your attacks and reactions to medications, and bring them in. Volunteer information about other drugs you're taking and other conditions you may have, if your doctor hasn't asked you already. They may have an impact on your migraine or interact with medications prescribed.

Because a doctor doesn't suggest these things, that doesn't mean the gates are closed, and if they are, push them open. If you don't like a treatment option, talk about that. If you're instructed to do something and didn't, explain why. If you're not sure why you're being asked to try something new, ask "How come?" If you get home and start wondering, Was it 1 or 2 milligrams, and was I supposed to take it before or after meals?, call. Don't wait for an appointment a month away to reveal a debilitating side effect or the fact that you've discontinued taking the drug. Take control outside the doctor's office. Once a drug has been prescribed, look it up in library books and periodicals, do a computer search, or purchase an up-to-date drug book. Find out all you can about it.

Tell your other doctors about your headache treatment plan so they're aware of any conflicts. Organize your medical and migraine records so they are orderly, accurate, and up to date. Keep track of your attacks in a headache diary or calendar. Record doses and treatment history, so you'll be as informed about your care as your physician in case of an emergency. Patients often don't express their concerns to their doctors, answering only those questions posed, accepting diagnoses and prescriptions without discussion, and keeping quiet about disagreements concerning their treatment, all because they don't want to be perceived as problem patients. Don't be silent. Ask questions and make suggestions. This is your health, your head, your migraine.

What kind of information should I record in a headache calendar or diary?

A headache diary is a thorough record that you keep each day, regardless of whether you've had a headache or not. Each day, record what you've eaten, your general emotional state, and key events that occurred during the day (e.g., conflicts). Make notes about how you slept the night before. On days that you have a headache, be sure to enter all the possible triggers (see the chart on page 197 to get you started). Keep the calendar for a minimum of two months—longer if you're having problems finding your triggers and if treatment is proving difficult.

If you don't normally keep a journal, maintaining this kind of record may seem like a big responsibility or an annoying chore. It can be both. It's also an essential step in most treatment plans, however, because patterns can emerge that target an approach to your migraine. Your efforts will be paid back in spades the first month you're migraine-free.

How do I rate my headaches?

You should rate your attacks on a scale from 1 to 5, or up through 10 if you feel you have that number of distinctly different attacks. Be very specific and descriptive about each level you've assigned. For instance, the definition of one patient's number 1 rating might be: "A throbbing that begins at the back of my neck and works forward. I can continue to work, and an OTC drug seems to take the worst of the pain away. In a few hours, it's gone." A number 5 rating could be described as "My skull and brain seem to expand and contract with each heartbeat, and the pressure makes it feel like my head will explode with each pulse. I can't work or do anything. I lie in a dark bedroom and throw up every hour. The pain lasts for at least a day." For the purposes of your headache diary or calendar, these definitions should apply only to *your* own headaches, not reflect some general "norm."

What are some medical insurance issues I might face?

In an ideal world, there would be none. Your migraine would be treated like any other serious disorder and your claims wouldn't be questioned. But in the current world of managed care and cutbacks in coverage, you may find that you have to appeal some decisions made by your medical insurance company. Write to complain if your claims are denied. Be sure you have your doctor's support and documentation. Politely persist, even if you're turned down again and again. Some insurance companies hope that complaints will go away if they're ignored, but give in when there's no sign that you're backing down. Once you've made that first inroad, subsequent claims will have a precedent to follow and may be more easily reimbursed.

How can I ensure that the cost of my treatment is covered?

Work within the rules of your plan. If a referral is needed by an in-network physician, go that route. If your HMO doesn't allow for a visit to a headache specialist without a referral and your primary care physician is being obstinate, switch to a new primary doctor who will work with you. When a specialist you prefer isn't on a particular plan, ask if he or she will consider joining, or lobby your employer to offer a choice of plans. If you have to pay the lion's share of medical costs, check to see what payment plans are available. There are often reasonable options, even if they're not offered voluntarily. Doctors usually want to help you; if you suggest a reasonable payment plan, they'll listen.

Or put the pressure on your medical insurance company. Write politely, but firmly, when requesting help, and enlist the support of your doctor's office. If the doctor's office or clinic is big enough, there might be a whole department dedicated to financial issues. Sometimes they'll act as your advocate in these difficult negotiations.

If, despite all efforts, your treatment isn't covered, really look at the math. Before you panic at the costs, review the long-term financial benefits. How much time and money are you losing each year to your battle with headache pain? What sacrifices is your family making now to accommodate your pain? How much do you spend each week on over-the-counter drugs? Compare that to the cost of a few visits to a specialist. Quality-of-life issues should enter the equation, too, even if they can't be measured in dollars.

EIGHT

Drug Therapy

CASE STUDY

On her first visit with me, Jen showed off the crowded entry under "Migraine" in her address book—seven names had been crossed out—and told me she hadn't had any luck with doctors or drugs in the past. She reeled off a long list of old prescriptions and claimed her bathroom cabinet was filled with enough over-the-counter NSAIDs to rival the local drugstore. But every treatment had failed, and as soon as it did, Jen had moved on to another physician.

I told Jen she might as well cross my name out, too, unless she was committed to sticking around even if initial efforts didn't work. The chances of our hitting her "magic bullet" on our first attempt were not high. I knew we'd find a medication plan to help her, but I explained that it might take time. Jen agreed to try. Over the next few months we tried a number of medicines, alone and in combination. One worked, but Jen's nausea became unbearable. I prescribed another that helped briefly. After a few weeks, though, the headaches came back.

We tried another one that worked on the pain but made her too drowsy. Jen was discouraged. I could tell she wondered, "Does he really know what he's doing?" But she stayed, because she liked my approach to migraine and because I answered all her questions, describing each drug and its effects in detail. After a while, Jen became more involved with the search herself. As we fine-tuned dosages, balancing

131

symptoms and side effects, she started asking questions and keeping notes on her reactions. She became more responsible about taking medications. When a drug failed, she remained optimistic about the next one's chances.

Eleven months after her first visit, we started to see real results. Jen was taking a preventive medication daily, but when a headache did show up, she took a second drug, Imitrex. If she felt nauseated or was vomiting, she added a third. Jen has been on this plan for four months now and can't believe the difference—her headaches come less often and don't cripple her like before. The bullet she was looking for isn't necessarily magic but it's working for her.

Migraine drugs have one goal—to bring relief from the symptoms of an attack, not the least of which is pain ranging from mild to murderous. There are a few ways drugs can do that: Some stop headaches from ever showing up. These drugs are called *prophylactics*, or preventives. Others alleviate the pain of an attack when one actually does arrive. Those are called everything from abortives, rescue drugs, and alleviatives, to relief drugs or acute medication. Finally, others target symptoms other than headache pain, such as migraine's terrible vomiting and nausea.

Now, take that list even further. Preventive drugs can be broken down into smaller categories of beta-blockers, calcium channel blockers, methysergide, and tricyclic antidepressants. The beta-blockers and calcium channel blockers work to prevent more mild attacks, while methysergide and the antidepressants help with more severe headaches. But once an attack rears its ugly head, preventives don't work. Then it's time for abortives. These cover the spectrum from over-the-counter drugs (called *analgesics*, or OTCs in migraine lingo), to ergotamines, to opioids and antidepressants. As you know, nonprescription drugs are the first rung on the ladder; they can often handle mild to moderate headaches. The next step up are analgesic products with caffeine added, then the ones with codeine. But the ergotamines, opioids and antidepressants are the big guns that you put to work when your headache looks severe. They can work wonders, but the side effects and possibility of addiction keep them from being a routine option. Some newer breakthrough medications, such as Imitrex (sumatriptan), don't fall neatly into any of these classifications yet. They seem to be in categories all of their own.

What do all those terms and names mean? They refer to the different ways the drugs work and their various agents —the basic ingredients of each. As you probably already know, the world of migraine drugs is filled with heavy-duty medical terminology. When these terms are explained, though, they're not so intimidating after all. It's easy for doctors to forget that their patients don't share a fascination for Latin, so remind your physician to speak English, spell out names for you, and tell you precisely what any unfamiliar terms mean. In a pinch, check the glossary in this book, but if you don't know what something means, make a doctor's appointment for the purpose of having a real live discussion that will address your particular concerns and questions about migraine drugs.

This chapter will help prepare you for that talk, by listing some of the drugs commonly discussed in the treatment of headache. Some are used for migraine, some for cluster headache, and others for tension-type headache. A few work on more than one type. Not all of these are drugs I recommend for my patients, but you may run across them in conversations with other sufferers. There may be others you've heard of that aren't here. That doesn't mean they may not be valid choices for you; ask your doctor why they are being prescribed. Furthermore, new medications are waiting for U.S. Food and Drug Administration (FDA) approval right now; soon you'll need to add them to this list, too. The inventory is flexible.

Here's how this list works: Medications are listed alphabetically by their generic names—the drug's main agent or the ingredient you're most likely to recognize. Under that you'll find the brand names it's sold under. In parentheses beside each brand is the name of the manufacturer, which might be helpful to you in the search for more information. The entries under each drug will provide a few basic facts about the medication. This information is far from complete. To do each drug justice, you will need a weighty tome like the latest edition of the *Physician's Desk Reference*, or its far more readable cousin, *The Pill Book*. These books, and other directories of drugs, can tell you far more about each medication. But both this list and those references are no substitute for a conversation with someone who has seen how these drugs work in real life—a headache specialist.

Even a catalog of side effects and potential drug conflicts you get from a doctor may not address your unique reactions. So you're the one in charge of monitoring your body's on-going response to each therapy. You need to watch for any signals that your body's not happy with the new drug—mental and physical changes only you might notice. Even if you just feel under the weather, let your doctor know. That way another person knowledgeable about possible side effects will be on the case.

Remember, this list is not the complete story! Draw up a string of questions for your doctor about these and other medicines you've heard about, built from the box below. Before you leave that physician's office, be sure you know exactly what it is that has been prescribed. Ask your doctor to write down the name for you on a sheet separate from the prescription—in clear capital letters, because the "myth" about doctor handwriting is sometimes only too true. Look for more information on your own.

Find out all you can before you take any drug, so you can make an informed judgment about your care. This list is just a beginning.

Note: Some drugs are called first-line defenses against migraine. That means they're FDA-approved for the treatment of migraine. Second-line defense drugs aren't approved by the FDA for migraine, but when migraineurs used them for the treatment of other conditions, they demonstrated an effect on headache pain, too. Some are being considered for front-line status. I feel strongly about using drugs that fall into the first two categories. Anything else, I would consider third-line medications, and they're questionable. Ask your doctor where your medication falls within those criteria, and why it's being prescribed for you now.

Questions to ask your physician about migraine drugs:

1. How can I tell which drug might work for me?
2. How long will it take to find the right one and the right dosage?
3. Is there a "smart" way to use this migraine medication?
4. Are there ways to make taking this drug easier?
5. Do all drugs lose their efficiency after you've been taking them awhile?
6. What forms does this medication come in? Is one more effective?
7. How long should I give each medicine before expecting results?
8. What drug interactions and combinations should I avoid?
9. What kind of medical history makes using this drug a bad idea?
10. What kind of side effects can I expect? Which should I report right away?
11. What are the risks with this treatment?
12. Can I become addicted to my painkiller?
13. What are the risks of long-term migraine drug use? What if I'm on this medication for the next ten years?
14. What does *that* word mean?

Generic name: acetaminophen
Tylenol (McNeil Pharmaceutical)
Acute medication: analgesic

An important first-line defense against migraine, acetaminophen is an effective abortive drug. It works on tension headaches as well as migraine and is a welcome option for those who can't tolerate aspirin. However, like all inexpensive, over-the-counter drugs, it's easy to abuse. Since no prescription is needed, patients give in to the need to take more than is recommended. So, one of this drug's potential side effects is rebound headache. Other effects include light-headedness and rash. Be alert for blood in your urine and reduced flow. Steer clear of alcohol while taking acetaminophen because it will upset your stomach. Excessive drinking while on this drug can cause permanent liver damage.

Generic name: acetaminophen, codeine
Tylenol with Codeine (McNeil Pharmaceutical)
Acute medication: analgesic/narcotic
  Tylenol with Codeine shares the same basic side effects and interactions as plain acetaminophen, but the addition of codeine introduces some new cautions. Patients needing a sleep aid to combat attacks are drawn to this compound version of acetaminophen. But with the addition of codeine it has added risks, including the potential for addiction. People with a history of drug and alcohol abuse should not take this compound. It also poses a danger for asthma patients and those with liver, kidney, or thyroid disease. Also, be aware that codeine contains a sulfite, which can be a migraine trigger.

Compound: acetaminophen, isometheptene mucate, dichloralphenazone
Midrin (Carnrick)
Acute medication: analgesic
  FDA-approved for the treatment of both migraine and tension headaches, this abortive is highly recommended. It works best when taken as soon as an attack is noticed. Its ingredients act as vasoconstrictors, muscle relaxers, and sedatives. Nursing mothers and people with stomach problems should use caution, and if you have glaucoma, kidney disease, hypertension, or porphyria, avoid this medication. Patients taking monoamine oxidase inhibitors (MAOs) should also steer clear. Dizziness and sleepiness are among reported side effects. Midrin is often prescribed for children, although for none younger than seven.

Generic name: amitriptyline
Elavil (Merck Sharp & Dohme)

Endep (Roche)
Preventive: tricyclic antidepressant

We're not quite sure why this drug works on migraine, but it does. Patients who have no symptoms of depression have gotten help with amitriptyline, so relief from those feelings can't be its only impact on migraine. Like other antidepressants, it is used as a preventive. One notable side effect is extreme sleepiness, which is not necessarily a bad thing if insomnia is one of your migraine symptoms. Less welcome are weight gain and constipation.

Generic name: aspirin or ASA
Bayer (Glenbrook)
Ecotrin enteric coated (SmithKline)
Acute or preventive medication: analgesic

The old standby. Most migraineurs are already aware that stomach problems are a risk with aspirin. So is sleeplessness. But other side effects to look out for are ringing in the ears and a feeling of dizziness. Rebound headaches from overuse are also common. Let your doctor know if you experience those. If you're already taking ibuprofen, don't add aspirin to your drug list; the combination raises the risk of stomach ulcers. Use a coated version of aspirin, such as Ecotrin, if you have stomach problems with this drug; it causes less upset. And do not give aspirin to migraineurs until they reach the age of sixteen, because of the risk of Reye's syndrome.

Compound: aspirin, acetaminophen, caffeine
Excedrin (Bristol-Myers)
Acute medication: analgesic

This compound combines two headache-busters, aspirin and acetaminophen, together with caffeine, which speeds their actions and prevents you from feeling sleepy. It may cause stomach irritation, so have something to eat when you take a dose. Beware of abuse with this drug, as with other OTCs. Ringing in your ears and a feeling of dizziness are some side effects. Anticoagulants should not be taken at the same time, nor should alcohol. Since this compound includes caffeine, cut down on the coffee and other caffeine sources while on this drug or you might get rebound headaches. Because it contains aspirin, which may cause Reye's syndrome in children, migraineurs under the age of sixteen should not take this medication.

Generic name: atenolol
Tenormin (ICI Pharmaceuticals)
Preventive medication: beta-blocker

This drug is primarily used to treat hypertension and some heart conditions. Some heart problems are worsened by this drug, however, so discuss its effects with your doctor. Diarrhea, dizziness, nausea, and changes in heart rate are among the side effects. Atenolol is a preventive that regulates blood flow and prostaglandins.

Generic name: butalbital
(There are several compounds that use this generic ingredient.)
Compound: butalbital, acetaminophen
Phrenilin, Phrenilin Forte (Carnrick)
Compound: butalbital, aspirin
Axotal (Adria)
Compound: butalbital, acetaminophen, caffeine
Fioricet (Sandoz)
Esgic, Esgic Plus (Forest)
Compound: butalbital, aspirin, caffeine
Fiorinal (Sandoz)
Compound: butalbital, codeine phosphate, aspirin, caffeine
Fiorinal with Codeine (Sandoz)
Acute medication: barbiturate

An abortive drug, butalbital relieves the pain of headache; other ingredients in the compounds act as sedatives and muscle relaxers. It is particularly effective on tension headaches, but shouldn't be used to treat chronic daily pain. There is a danger of abuse with these compounds, so monitor your doses carefully, never using more than prescribed. Dizziness or sleepiness are common side effects, so avoid activities that require you to be alert, such as driving. Watch for any changes in your mental and physical condition and report them to your doctor.

Fiorinal is an analgesic combined with a barbiturate and has more potential side effects than the other compounds; discuss these with your physician. Avoid drinking alcohol when taking this medication, or you risk overdose. If you have a bone marrow or liver condition called porphyria, or have a history of depression or drug abuse, do not use this drug. Women who are pregnant or planning a pregnancy should stay away from these compounds, as should breast-feeding mothers. Kidney and liver damage are a result of overuse, plus rebound headaches. Butalbital interacts with many other drugs, so be sure to discuss any medications you're currently taking—prescription and OTC—with your doctor. Some of the milder compounds are okay for kids, but be aware that they'll induce sleep.

Generic name: butorphanol tartrate
Stadol (Bristol Labs)
Acute medication: opioid
This abortive drug, FDA-approved for migraine, is similar to methadone, and has been found to be quite effective in the management of migraine pain. It also acts as a sedative. This drug should not be used when there has been a head injury or if heart and lung problems are present. Nursing mothers and pregnant women are advised to stay away, as are elderly patients. Be alert for signs of nausea, dizziness, ringing in the ears, changes in heart rate and breathing problems. Stadol's status as a controlled substance is being debated in some states.

Generic name: chlorpromazine
Thorazine (SmithKline Beecham)
Acute medication: dopamine antagonist/antiemetic
This drug is a powerful mood regulator. It is sometimes classified as the antinausea medication phenothiazine, along with prochlorperazine and metoclorpramide. It has effects on the nausea and vomiting that accompany migraine. Muscle spasms are a frequently noted side effect and can become permanent. Other effects range throughout the spectrum of seriousness, so ask your doctor to tell you more. Negative interactions with other drugs are also a problem, so be sure to learn what to avoid. Do not take antacids or drink alcohol while on this drug.

Generic name: clonidine hydrochloride
Catapres (Boehringer-Ingelhelm)

The benefits of this drug have not been proven; it seems to have more of a placebo effect than anything else. Its primary use is as a treatment for high blood pressure, among other conditions. It has some serious side effects, however, such as depression and insomnia. Users with hypertension, kidney and liver disease, a history of heart attack, or porphyria should certainly avoid it. It has been found to have a place in the treatment of childhood migraine and cluster headache.

Generic name: cyproheptadine
Periactin (Merck Sharp & Dohme)
Preventive medication: antiserotonin/antihistamine

This drug is often found effective when treating children with migraine attacks. With adults, its use is more problematic because it causes drowsiness and can lead to excessive weight gain if taken for a long time. It's generally limited to use with stubborn or chronic migraine.

Generic name: dexamethasone
Decadron Tablets (Merck Sharp & Dohme)
Acute or preventive medication: corticosteroid

If your headache lasts longer than seventy-two hours, you may be given this powerful drug. It's primarily used to treat a number of other disorders, including arthritis, allergies, and asthma. Ask your doctor about its many side effects. Use with caution and stick to the lowest possible dose.

Generic name: dexamethasone acetate
Dalalone D.P. (Forest)
Decadron-LA (Merck Sharp & Dohme)

These two drugs share the same properties as dexamethasone. See the preceding entry.

Generic name: diazepam
Valium (Wyeth-Ayerst)
Preventive medication: tranquilizer

In the past, this drug was often used to treat migraine associated with anxiety triggers. Nowadays, its use is limited in migraine treatment because of the risk of dependency. Side effects include coordination problems, weakness, depression, and feelings of light-headedness. Some newer therapeutic drugs, such as Atavan, are shorter acting, so may become more popular than Valium for migraine treatment.

Generic name: dihydroergotamine mesylate
DHE-45 (or **D.H.E. 45**) (Sandoz)
Acute medication: ergotamine/antiserotonin (serotonin antagonist)

This drug, FDA-approved for migraine, is generally used for the treatment of headaches that are severe and unmanageable. DHE-45 is given by shot (intramuscular injection, or IM) or taken through intravenous drip (IV), usually performed in hospitals or a doctor's office. It is effective on severe headaches, even when taken well into an attack. It also works on acute cluster headaches. Unlike other ergots, it is not habit-forming and doesn't normally cause nausea or vomiting. Some patients take metoclopramide before the DHE if they find they do get nausea. It has many of the same side effects as ergots, described under that entry. Like those other ergots, it's not for patients who have the following conditions: liver and kidney problems, coronary artery disease and other vascular disorders, bacterial infections, and women who are or are trying to become pregnant. Rebound headaches are a danger with overuse. Currently, DHE for migraine only has been approved as an injection, but look for FDA approval of a nasal-spray version soon (see also ergotamine.)

Generic name: divalproex sodium, valproic acid and sodium valproate
Depakote (Abbott)
Preventive medication: anticonvulsant/therapeutic

FDA-approved for migraine, this is an epilepsy and seizure medication long used for migraine treatment as well. New studies confirm its effectiveness on migraine and cluster headaches, with a success rate of up to 75 percent. It has generally replaced the use of phenytoin, another anticonvulsant sold under the brand name Dilantin. Like prednisone, it regulates sleep patterns that have an effect on migraine. It should not be given to children, however, since it increases their risk for hepatitis. Side effects include feelings of weakness and fatigue, as well as mood changes. Users may gain weight despite loss of appetite. Stomach upset is common. Carefully monitor your liver functions with your doctor while on this medication. It's a preventive medication and can't relieve a headache already in progress.

Generic name: ergotamine tartrate
Ergostat (Parke-Davis)
Ergomar (Fisons)
Medihaler Ergotamine
Compound: ergotamine tartrate, caffeine
Cafergot (Sandoz)
Wigraine (Organon)
Compound: ergotamine tartrate, pentobarbital, Bellafoline
Bellergal (Sandoz)
Acute medication (except for Bellergal, which is preventive): antiserotonin

One of the benefits of ergotamine is that it's available in so many different forms: Ergostat and Ergomar are sublingual tablets (taken under the tongue); Medihaler is a mouth spray; Cafergot is a rectal suppository; Wigraine is taken as a tablet, as is Bellergal-S. We're still not sure exactly how ergotamine works on migraine, but it performs a number of functions that relate to the suspected causes of headache pain. It can constrict blood vessels. It also regulates levels of serotonin. Ergots are often used to treat cluster headaches as well as migraine. Since the drug is available in virtually every form, from shots (DHE) to inhalers, ask your doctor which will work faster and more effectively than others for you.

About 10 percent of patients have terrible attacks of vomiting or nausea while on ergots. They tend to treat that symptom with an additional drug like metoclopramide. A brief period of unusually rapid or slow heartbeat has been noted as a side effect. Some patients report feeling weak in the knees, and having a numb or tingling sensation in their feet and hands. If feet and hands become cold and pale as well as numb, or you experience muscle pain, then you should consult a doctor immediately about overdosing. This is not the kind of drug you should be using every day, even in low doses. Improper use can lead to serious results. Avoid using ergots if you have a bacterial infection, coronary artery disease, vascular disorders, kidney or liver problems, or if you're planning to become pregnant. It's not for hemiplegic migraine.

You can become dependent on ergots. Withdrawal brings more headaches and nausea, so be sure your doctor is monitoring your dosages and that you're both on the alert for addiction symptoms. Some forms of Cafergot may be difficult to find now; the manufacturer has stated the intention of discontinuing some of its line. (See also DHE-45.)

Generic name: fenophrophen
Nalfon (Dista)
Acute medication: NSAID
This abortive medication soothes inflamed blood vessels, cutting down on blood flow. If you have nausea and vomiting, NSAIDs are not appropriate medications. Sudden onset of interior bleeding and ulcers are a real risk with this drug, so be sure your doctor is monitoring you closely. Side effects can range from blurred vision, constipation, and nausea to others rarer but far more serious. Discuss potential effects with your doctor prior to use.

Generic name: flunarizine
Sibelium
Preventive medication: calcium channel blocker
This vasoconstrictor is available only in Europe.

Generic name: gabapentin
Neurontin (Parke-Davis)
Preventive medication: anticonvulsant
This drug is new on the scene and looks promising for the treatment of migraine. Developed for chronic pain care, it was originally approved for use against seizures. Because it is so new, ask your doctor about the latest information on side effects and interactions.

Generic name: fluoxetine
Prozac (Lilly)
Preventive medication: antidepressant

Prozac's effects on headache were first spotted by migraineurs who were taking the drug to treat other conditions, such as depression, guilt feelings, obsessive-compulsive disorders, weight problems, or chronic pain. But Prozac can also create feelings of nervousness, anxiety, or fatigue. Be alert for stomach upset, too. Combining this drug with MAOs can lead to fatal consequences, so use extreme caution. If you're taking anticoagulants to prevent clotting, Prozac is not a good choice, either. Side effects are legion, so consult with your doctor before use. Stay away from alcohol while taking Prozac; it contributes to depression and can have a toxic reaction with the drug.

Generic name: ibuprofen
Advil (Whitehall)
Medipren (McNeil Consumer Products)
Motrin (Upjohn)
Nuprin (Bristol-Myers)
Rufen (Boots)
Acute medication: NSAID

In addition to combating headache pain, this nonprescription drug aids in the treatment of menstrual cramps, inflammation, and arthritis. It reduces sensitivity to light in patients who don't have aura. It also works very well in the treatment of menstrual migraine. Take it with food to prevent stomach problems, and stay away from alcohol. If you're also taking aspirin, the combination can lead to stomach ulcers, so don't mix these two OTC drugs. If you get symptoms like sleeplessness, tiredness, dizziness, or depression, stop using ibuprofen. Other side effects to watch for include diarrhea and constipation. Ironically, too much of this drug can cause headaches. If you get chills, numbness in your feet or hands, or notice blood in the toilet, see a doctor. Do not use NSAIDs if symptoms include nausea and vomiting. Finally, stick to recommended doses—overuse leads to dependency and rebound headaches.

Generic name: indomethacin
Indocin (Merck Sharp & Dohme)
Acute or preventive medication: NSAID

This antiinflammatory blocks the production of prostaglandins and therefore regulates blood flow through vessels. It's an abortive medication that is primarily used to treat arthritis and other kinds of joint pain. It's used on exertional and orgasmic migraine. Do not take Indocin if vomiting and nausea are present. Ulcers and interior bleeding can occur suddenly, so be sure to see your doctor regularly for monitoring.

Generic name: isocarboxazid
Marplan (Roche)
Preventive medication: monoamine oxidase inhibitor (MAO)/antidepressant

A medication to treat depression, this MAO is also used as a preventive for migraine. Side effects include blurred vision, dizziness or lightheadedness, sleepiness, hunger, and the sweats. Sexual appetite might be affected. When taking this medication, you must remove all foods with tyramine from your diet, or interaction can be severe—even fatal. Get a list of these foods from your doctor: some examples include avocados, bean curd, beer, ale, caviar, cheese, figs, dried fish, liver, some dairy products, some meats, soups with protein extracts, soy sauce, and dietary supplements such as Marmite. This MAO is not considered a first line of defense and is best reserved for chronic pain.

Generic name: ketoprofen
Orudis (Wyeth-Ayerst)
Acute medication: NSAID

Another antiinflammatory. It should not be used when you have vomiting and nausea. As with other NSAIDs, beware of rebound headaches from overuse. Common side effects include kidney problems, constipation and diarrhea, depression, insomnia, and vision problems, among others. If you've had problems taking aspirin, let your doctor know, because this has similar effects.

Generic name: ketorolac tromethamine (IM)
Toradol (Syntex)
Acute medication: NSAID

A shot of this drug works on acute migraine and is sometimes used in emergency-room care. Patients may need to take an antinausea medication first. It's a potent drug, so be sure to learn its side effects and interactions.

Generic name: lidocaine
Xylocaine (Astra)
Acute medication

Lidocaine is considered an "urgent care" medication, which means it's not really for use at home, but rather in a hospital or clinic. That's because it is administered through drops dripped into the nose steadily over a period of half a minute, while the patient lies down with his or her head tilted in the direction of headache pain. Lidocaine has been around for awhile and is also used for cluster headaches. It is believed that lidocaine numbs the nerves behind the eyes, reducing the pain and sensitivity to light. Nausea also goes away. Side effects include irritation in the nasal passages. More studies are being done, but for now this drug is still not approved by the FDA for the treatment of migraine. Consequently, it's not considered a first-line medication.

Generic name: lithium carbonate
Eskalith (SmithKline Beecham)
Lithane (Miles Pharmaceutical)
Preventive medication: antidepressant/antimanic/anticonvulsant

Lithium is not used for migraine but to treat disorders, like cluster headaches, that present a regular cycle. For cluster, it is used as a rescue medication when ergots and verapamil fail to stop a cycle. Lithium has an effect on the hypothalamus and therefore on sleep patterns that affect migraine.

Generic name: meperidine hydrochloride
Demerol (Winthrop)
Acute medication: narcotic analgesic

Use caution with this abortive drug. You should not use

it during the two weeks before, after, or during treatment with antidepressant MAOs such as Nardil. Even users who don't experience this dangerous combination can expect side effects like nausea, sleepiness, vomiting, and sweats. Other effects exist, and dependency is a risk as well, so learn more about this drug and use caution before taking it.

Generic name: methadone
Dolophine (Lilly)
Acute medication: narcotic

This potentially addictive drug is usually given only in cases of very severe pain. Discuss the size of your dose; doctors generally prefer a dose large enough to cover the entire span of the headache, so another is not needed. Multiple doses only add to the risk of addiction.

Generic name: methysergide
Sansert *(Sandoz)*
Preventive medication: antiserotonin antagonist/ergot type

This drug was the first medication to be approved by the FDA specifically for the treatment of migraine. Nowadays, reports of side effects and the introduction of Imitrex (sumatriptan) have reduced the number of users, and doctors are increasingly reluctant to prescribe it. However, it is sometimes still used as a defense against migraine with aura. It is usually administered in a hospital setting where its effects can be monitored closely. Side effects include insomnia, mood swings, hallucinations, nausea, vomiting, diarrhea, and more serious problems such as chest pains, heart and lung problems, and urinary tract blocks.

Because accumulation of this drug can be toxic, you should use it for no more than four to six months at a time, then take a drug holiday of two months before resuming treatment. Gradually take yourself off the drug, however, or you might get rebound headaches. If you are careful to maintain this cycle, you should avoid the more serious side effects connected to its use. It is a preventive medication that has an effect on serotonin levels. It is no longer favored for the treatment of cluster headache unless it's used to treat the first few attacks. It's not a good choice for young patients with cluster; for them, side effects become more intense.

Generic name: metoclopramide hydrochloride
Reglan (A.H. Robins)
Acute medication: antiemetic/dopamine antagonist

An antinausea medication, this drug is used when vomiting and nausea are symptoms of an attack. It's also taken in combination with other medications that have stomach upset as a side effect. It may not be suitable for young sufferers.

Generic name: metoprolol
Lopressor (Geigy)
Preventive medication: beta-blocker

A preventive medication, Lopressor uses blockers to cut down on prostaglandins and reduce the width of arteries. It is not to be used in combination with ergots. Side effects range from fatigue to slow pulse rates to cold hands and feet. Asthma patients should stay away from beta-blockers.

Generic name: nadolol
Corgard (Bristol Myers-Squibb)
Preventive medication: beta-blocker

Intended for the treatment of high blood pressure and some heart problems, this drug prevents arteries and blood vessels from dilating; I have found it to be very effective on migraine. Dosing should be routine, and on no account should two doses be taken at once. Beware of the risks for heart attack, and closely monitor changes in your mental and physical condition.

Generic name: naproxen sodium
Aleve (TK)
Anaprox (Syntex)
Acute or preventive medication: NSAID

A popular OTC option, this medication is effective and less expensive than prescription treatments. Like other OTC medications, it's often used as a "rescue drug" when your prescription medication doesn't kick in. Some people have reported success using it to relieve their cyclic headaches. It's an abortive medication that works particularly well for menstrual migraine; sufferers can time doses for the days just before and after a period. Watch for side effects common to other OTC medicines, such as stomach upset. If you're having trouble sleeping or feel tired and depressed, it could be due to this medicine. Ironically, headaches are a side effect experienced when it's taken too often, as a result of the rebound effect. So beware of dependency and overuse. More serious side effects, such as numbness in the hands or feet, chills, or blood in the stool, are not too common, but should be reported to a doctor right away. Avoid alcohol and aspirin when taking this drug, because of increased risk of severe stomach problems. Antacids can cut down on naproxen's effectiveness, so don't take them at the same time. This drug may be prescribed for children, with dosage based on weight.

Generic name: naproxen
Naprosyn (Syntex)
Acute or preventive medication: NSAID

This basic naproxen shares the same properties as naproxen sodium, so see the preceding entry.

Generic name: nifedipine
Adalat (Miles Pharmaceutical)
Procardia (Pfizer Labs Division)
Procardia XL (Pfizer Labs Division)
Preventive medication: calcium channel blocker

The beneficial effects of this medication add up over time, and are felt only after a few weeks of treatment. Unfortunately, that delayed reaction causes some users to give up on this medication too soon. Some notes for users: Adalat is used only occasionally. Let your dentist know you're using this drug before getting work performed. Ask about interactions with other drugs—there are several to avoid, like beta-blockers. Low blood pressure is one side effect; ask about others that range in levels of seriousness.

Generic name: nimodine
Nimotop (Miles)
Preventive medication: calcium channel blocker

Although primarily for treatment of ruptured blood vessels, this occasionally can be a very effective migraine therapy. This drug's agent is so tiny it is able to cross the blood–brain barrier and really target migraine pain. Monitor blood pressure since low levels are one of the few potential side effects. Unfortunately this drug is still quite expensive.

Generic name: nortriptyline
Pamelor (Sandoz)
Preventive medication: tricyclic antidepressant

A less sedating alternative to amitriptyline. Patients have reported a wide range of side effects while on this drug, ranging in seriousness from rashes to risk of heart attack. Because of the number of effects and their range, report any change in your physical and mental state to your physician while you are on this drug.

Generic name: phenelzine or phenylzine sulfate
Nardil (Parke-Davis)
Preventive medication: antidepressant/monoamine oxidase inhibitor (MAO)

This prophylactic is not a first choice because its serious risk factors often outweigh its benefits. When combined with some foods, such as cheddar cheese, this drug can be fatal. Discuss possible side effects with your doctor.

Generic name: pizotifen
Sandomigran (Sandoz)
Preventive medication: serotonin antagonist/antihistamine

This drug is not currently available in the U.S., although it can be found in Canada and some European countries. Weight gain and drowsiness are known side effects; less common ones include muscle pain, depression, anxiety, dizziness, impotence, and rebound headaches. Avoid drinking alcohol while taking it. Pregnant and breast-feeding women should not use this drug, nor should patients with urinary tract conditions, closed-angle glaucoma, or kidney problems.

Generic name: prednisone
Deltasone (Upjohn)
Acute medication for cluster, preventive medication for severe migraine

A heavy hitter, this drug is brought in only after others have failed in cluster headache treatment because its side effects are so severe. This drug has a tremendous impact on the immune system, so users should be monitored carefully for infection both while taking it and during withdrawal. It can also cause mental problems. Weight gain, mood swings, and insomnia are other pitfalls of this medication.

Generic name: prochlorperazine
Compazine (SmithKline & French)
Acute medication: antiemetic

Although this drug can be used to treat the nausea and vomiting of migraine, as well as its anxiety-producing effects, it can have serious side effects. Some, like muscle twitches, can become permanent. Use with caution, and discuss the risks thoroughly with your doctor.

Generic name: promazine hydrochloride
Sparine (Wyeth-Ayerst)
Acute medication: antiemetic

This medication allows doctors to treat both the headache and nausea or vomiting at the same time. It's non-habit-forming. An added benefit in some cases is that it acts as a sedative, bringing the sleep that speeds recovery. Of course, some patients may want to avoid a medicine that causes drowsiness. Low blood pressure is counted as the downside; patients need constant intake of fluids, meaning that it is more often administered in hospitals where IVs can be given.

Generic name: propranolol
Inderal (Wyeth-Ayerst)
Inderal-LA (Wyeth-Ayerst)
Preventive medication: beta-blocker

FDA-approved for migraine, many migraineurs use this prophylactic for their headache treatment, which is really for the treatment of a number of heart-related conditions. It works on both migraine with aura and migraine without; about 70 percent of patients who use it get less severe attacks on propranolol. Side effects range from fatigue, cramping, enhanced dreams, and ringing in the ears to depression, heart block, and short-term memory loss. Check with your doctor about drug interactions and risk of heart attack. Do not use at the same time as ergots.

Generic name: sertraline
Zoloft (Pfizer-Roerig Pratt)
Preventive medication: antidepressant

This drug is close to Prozac in its action and is very popular now for the treatment of depression. It is prescribed more often than Prozac because it works faster and leaves the body more quickly than the other drug. Because of that speedy action, its side effects are fewer than those of Prozac. For these reasons, it's also becoming more popular for migraine treatment. Do not use this drug in combination with MAOs; the results can be very serious. The most common side effects include diarrhea, nausea, and stomach upset. Patients may experience feelings of weakness, tiredness, or confusion. Some men report problems in ejaculating. Less common side effects run the gamut from bad breath to hallucinations, so consult your doctor if you notice any mental or physical changes when on this drug.

Generic name: steroids

Steroids are sometimes prescribed in the treatment of cluster headaches, and they're an essential treatment for temporal arteritis, a rare form of migraine found most often in older patients. Unfortunately, side effects can be extreme, among them excessive weight gain and increased risk of osteoporosis. Steroid use is very habit-forming. There are many dangers inherent in this treatment, so discuss this option with your doctor and find out more.

Generic name: sumatriptan, sumatriptophen
Imitrex (Cerenex)
Acute medication: vasoconstrictor

FDA-approved for migraine, sumatriptan is one of the newest and most effective medications for migraine. About 70 percent of patients taking the injection—even those with severe migraine—report that they get relief in about an hour. You may hear it referred to as 5-HT1, which means it is related to serotonin. Sumatriptan also works by reducing the number of chemicals that signal blood vessels to widen. An abortive medication, it is taken when headache pain first makes itself known, but can also stop a headache that's well under way. It also helps with the headache hangover so many patients experience after pain is gone. It might be effective on cluster headaches, too, but has not yet been FDA-approved as a treatment for that.

As a vasoconstrictor, it should be avoided by people at risk for heart problems, high blood pressure, or hypertension—especially smokers. Older sufferers should also be cautious about using Imitrex unless the potential for heart disease, diabetes, and hypertension have been ruled out, and children should not use this drug. Do not use this medication at the same time you're using ergots or DHE. Basilar or hemiplegic migraine sufferers should not use this drug.

Side effects reported include mild forms of the following: tingling sensations, a feeling of pressure in the chest, flushed skin, a feeling of spreading warmth, dizziness, weakness, and a stiff neck. Skin irritation at the site of the injection is common. If these effects don't pass quickly, inform your doctor. Rebound headaches have been reported in some cases. Migraineurs are excited about a nasal spray version, which will work faster than tablets and will be a welcome alternative for those who find it hard to inject themselves.

Generic name: timolol
Blocadren (Merck Sharp & Dohme)
Preventive medication: beta-blocker

Like other beta-blocker preventatives, this medication, which is FDA-approved for migraine, constricts arteries and cuts down on prostaglandins. This is a preventive medication. Avoid this drug if you're using an ergot-based medication, including DHE. When used with calcium channel blockers it increases your risk of cardiac problems, and when taken with NSAIDs, the effectiveness of both drugs is reduced. People with persistent low blood pressure and heart problems should use caution with this medication. Watch for changes in pulse rate and signs of fatigue. Other side effects include breathing problems, cold hands and feet, loss of sexual appetite, chest pain, and changes in pulse rate. It shouldn't be used by asthma patients or children.

Generic name: trimethobenzamide
Tigan (Beecham)
Acute medication: antiemetic

This is a mild antinausea medication that is particularly good for children whose migraine attacks are accompanied by stomach upset and vomiting. However, be alert for signs of fatigue, low blood pressure, blurred vision, and muscle cramps. Patients may also feel dizzy or confused while on this medication.

Generic name: verapamil
Calan (Searle)
Isoptin (Knoll)
Verelan (Lederle; Wyeth-Ayerst)
Preventive medication: calcium channel blocker

This preventive is the calcium channel blocker of choice for migraine. It works on cluster headache, too. A single dose each day is preferred. Do not use this drug, however, if you have consistently low blood pressure, sick sinus syndrome, heart block, or Wolff-Parkinson White syndrome. Constipation is the side effect most often reported. The few others include nausea and dizziness.

Generic name: tramadol
Ultram
Acute medication: opioid

This has only recently become available in the U.S., and many doctors are still reluctant to prescribe it since seizures have been reported among some migraine users. Nausea and vomiting are more common side effects; users are wise to take this in combination with an antiemetic. Other effects include dizziness, sleepiness, constipation, and sometimes headache. Do not use this drug with alcohol or if you're taking MAOs. If you've had a head injury, have lung problems, or stomach conditions, also avoid the use of this medication.

NINE

Alternatives to Drug Treatment for Migraine

CASE STUDY

Sarah had her first migraine attack in her stress-filled senior year of college. She remembers lying in bed, praying for the pain to stop, and wondering what was wrong with her. Although she didn't get aura, Sarah did get sick, vomiting several times during the attack. She had no idea what hit her. Later, some friends told Sarah she'd just had her first migraine. For a few years, she tried using over-the-counter drugs, but the attacks started showing up more often. Finally, she saw a doctor. Several doctors. Some didn't take her seriously. Nothing the others prescribed seemed to help. One physician put her on DHE-45 injections, but, as Sarah put it, "There was just no way. I tried, but every time he got near my skin with that needle, I just couldn't face it." Sarah didn't tell the doctor about her problem—she was too embarrassed to let on that she was afraid of needles and that taking such a powerful drug made her nervous. Instead, she said, "I was popping two, three, four Excedrin as soon as I felt a headache coming on. I kept a bottle in my briefcase. Then I had one really bad attack. I remember thinking, if I don't get relief soon, I don't know what I'll do." Sarah was still afraid to talk to her doctor (a signal to look for another one!) so she asked around for advice. Even though she really didn't think it would work, Sarah began taking a daily dose of two leaves of an herb called feverfew, because a friend was using it. Finally, she switched doctors and visited the clinic. The feverfew had taken two months to kick in, but by that time there was no question that she was feeling better. The headaches didn't come as often, and when they did, the pain was manageable. Like many doctors, I'm reluctant to recommend herbal remedies, but I could see the herb was bringing Sarah relief. I suggested she try another nondrug therapy, biofeedback, as well. She's now being trained in that and enjoys the sense of control it gives her. But, in the meantime, she says, "Feverfew is working for me right now. I figure it buys me time to look for other things that will help, too. That's good enough for me after all those years of pain."

Today there are more options for treating migraine than ever before, giving new hope to sufferers who have lived with pain for years. But even as the number of drugs used to treat migraine increases, many patients are turning to drug-free alternative treatments for relief—folk remedies and technological advances that run the gamut from traditional tonics and meditation, through acupuncture, massage, and aromatherapy, to biofeedback and routine exercise.

Often these alternatives are an important part of a sufferer's treatment plan. For some, the cost of maintaining a drug therapy is prohibitive, especially if health insurance isn't available. For others, the idea of taking drugs is distasteful for various reasons. Many migraineurs experience side effects that make drugs a choice between the lesser of two evils: headache pain or punishing symptoms from the medication itself. Other people may not be able to take the drug that works for them because it interferes with treatments they're taking for other conditions. Pregnant women who are unable to take medication often find relief through alternative therapies, although they should avoid some herbal remedies as well.

For most migraineurs, however, options like the ones described in this chapter are simply used to augment an ongoing drug treatment plan—bringing added relief from the pain, alleviating some symptoms, or preventing stress triggers from taking hold. These migraineurs want to use every possible means at their disposal for battling their headaches. In fact, about one in four people in the United States who suffer from chronic pain use some combination of conventional therapy and nondrug alternatives in their treatment. A decade ago most doctors would have scorned the use of folk remedies, but a survey conducted in 1993 showed that as many as 70 percent of family doctors were now open to the suggestion of alternatives for their patients. That's quite a change. Many doctors are aware that the most modern pharmaceutical treatments use the same basic ingredients as ancient folk remedies.

Keep in mind that the jury is still out on many of the treatments outlined in this chapter. Some, such as biofeedback and relaxation techniques, are universally acknowledged to help in the treatment of migraine. Virtually any specialist will discuss those options with a headache patient. Other treatments, such as herbal remedies, hypnosis, and acupuncture, remain the subject of controversy. For every anecdotal story in favor of these treatments there is another where it was ineffective—but the same is true even with drug treatments. We've all heard about someone who was treated with Coca Cola and an aspirin; it sounds great, but that's only one person. Migraine is highly individual and so is its treatment.

Most drug-free alternatives, though, fall into the gray area between those extremes. Sufferers spread the word that a therapy works, building to a high tally of anecdotal reports that tends to add weight to the claims—even though the therapy's effectiveness may not be widely documented in medical studies. The trick for migraineurs is to approach these nondrug options with the same caution and concerns they bring to any of their prescription treatments. Use your own careful judgment and get professional advice when exploring any alternatives.

Remember, too, that some people react to *any* new migraine therapy with a brief remission of pain. Doctors call this the *placebo response*—the enthusiasm of a patient for a new treatment has a physiological effect as well as a psychological one. For a brief period the mind convinces the body that the treatment is working. That may account for some of the positive reactions people have had to even the wackiest alternative treatments. Back in prehistoric days, treatments included removing sections of the skull in a highly risky surgery called trepanning. Later, sufferers claimed they got relief by wrapping their heads in the rope used to hang a criminal or used in a suicide; by arranging matches in a special pattern on their foreheads; by rubbing affected areas with a live toad; or by sleeping with scissors under their pillows. Remedies have come and gone through the years, some far more rational than these, others even more absurd.

Obviously, most of the alternatives people explore today aren't nearly that bizarre. But charlatans still exist, pedaling reasonable-sounding "cures" to migraineurs who are desperate for relief. So keep an open mind, but get all the information you can before trying a new treatment. Most people are best off if they take a multidisciplined approach to treating their migraine, including drug treatment, biofeedback, physical therapy of some kind, a few lifestyle changes, and perhaps some of the options mentioned in the following pages. As long as those alternative treatments don't conflict with other therapies already in progress, they can be an effective part of the migraine plan.

An English friend of mine told me to try feverfew. What is it?

Feverfew is an herbal remedy long known to migraine sufferers in England. It does not abort headaches already in progress but may work as a preventive. Feverfew, sometimes used as a sedative or gentle laxative, is derived from plants in the chrysanthemum family. Its botanical name is *Tanacetum parthenium,* and the plant bears small, daisylike white flowers. Herbal teas made from the dried leaves of these plants can be found in health food stores in the United States, under the name of feverfew or more generic names like "Headache Remedy." Advocates claim that feverfew works by cutting down on the supply of serotonin, reducing the severity of attacks, or preventing migraine attacks altogether. The herb may also help soothe inflamed blood vessels in the brain, relieving the intense pressure suffered by many migraineurs. Recent studies have found a chemical agent called a *pathenolide* that might be the key to feverfew's reputation as a migraine treatment. More needs to be discovered about this herb before doctors begin to "prescribe" it for their migraine patients. In the meantime, though, many patients report beneficial effects after two or more months of daily dosages.

Do herbs like feverfew really work?

The question really is, "Will feverfew work for *you*?" As with other migraine treatments, response to feverfew and other herbal remedies varies by individual. Some researchers think feverfew acts as a placebo—belief in the herb's effects is so strong that force of will, rather than the herb itself, is causing the positive effects. In reality, there may be just the *perception* of a positive effect. Others argue that the herbal remedy's effectiveness is just temporary. However, feverfew was found more effective than prescription drug treatments in two clinical trials performed in the United Kingdom in the 1980s. Patients reported everything from partial to total relief. The results of these studies prompted the Canadian Health and Welfare Department to approve sale of the herb for migraine prevention in their own country. In the clinical trials, patients received a daily dose equal to about two medium-sized leaves of the herb.

How do you take herbal remedies like feverfew?

Most patients take feverfew in capsule form. Others use the dried leaves in a tea, which is often referred to in herbal literature as an *infusion*. The trouble with the capsules and teas most commonly found in the United States is that the size or concentration of the dose may not be revealed on the label. Strength varies from tea to tea, so you may have to try several brands before finding one that is effective. Many people report having to take more capsules than the suggested dose on the package label. Fresh leaves appear to be the most effective, but generally these are only available in the spring and summer. Fresh leaves can be eaten; their bitter taste needs some masking, so they are best disguised with other greens in a salad or sandwich. Some people get painful mouth sores from eating the fresh herb, so be on the alert for an outbreak of canker sores in your mouth or on your tongue. Naturally, you should inform your physician about this or any other herbal treatments you explore.

Can meadowsweet help?

Meadowsweet is an age-old remedy, but many modern sufferers also proclaim the benefits of this plant. Meadowsweet bark contains salicylate, which is one of the basic components of aspirin, so it's not so surprising that this herb is considered an effective remedy. Fans point to the fact that dosing with the herb has none of the side effects of taking aspirin and, in fact, combats the stomach upset that aspirin can produce. Other plants with salicyclate are white willow, also known as *Salix alba*, and black poplar (*Populus nigra*). Meadowsweet is perhaps the one more often found in stores offering folk remedies. Weak teas made from this plant's leaves should be taken three times each day. The tannins in the herb also help with the nausea and stomach pain of a migraine attack. Remember, if your headaches don't respond to herbal treatments, you shouldn't discount the modern equivalents, such as aspirin, made from similar components. Drugs may offer more controlled or concentrated amounts of the basic substances than these herbs and may be processed more efficiently by some sufferers.

What other kinds of herbs combat migraine pain?

Chamomile, lemon balm, and passionflower are considered by many to be useful antiinflammatory treatments. They work to alleviate headache pain once it strikes, rather than prevent it. Because chamomile is such a popular tea, it is perhaps the most accessible herbal treatment. Most supermarkets carry versions of chamomile tea made from the leaves of the plant. There are two varieties of chamomile, Roman and German, both of which have similar properties. Chamomile has been reported to aid women with painful menstruation, so this herb may be of double use for women who started taking birth control pills to cut back on period pain but then found that the pill triggered migraine.

Lemon balm is another herb with a nonmedicinal taste that makes it popular with nonsufferers as well as people with migraine. For treatment of headaches, three cups of tea made from the plant's leaves should be taken as a daily dose. Chamomile and lemon balm have the added benefit of soothing the stomach upset that accompanies migraine attacks. Both are also available as oils for use in aromatherapy.

Passiflora incarnata is the botanical term for passionflower; teas infused from the roots of this plant are used to promote relaxation and make migraineurs drowsy enough to sleep. Pregnant women are often warned against this herb, though, because it's thought passionflower affects the muscles of the womb. Drink passionflower tea three times a day, or just before bedtime if you're using it to help you sleep.

Evening primrose oil has also cropped up as a pain reliever in discussions among migraineurs. Mint teas and evening primrose oil have been known to help some people. Betony may have an effect on tension headaches, may combat stress, and may be used as a sleep aid when taken in a tea made from the plant's leaves and stems. Other herbs that target stress are damiana, valerian, and vervain. Large doses of valerian can reverse its effects, however, and make a person excitable instead of relaxed. People report luck with teas made from parsley, sage, rosemary, and thyme, as well as basil, lavender, ginger, and catnip. But just how easily some of those are swallowed is another question!

Should children be given herbal remedies?

Herbal remedies can be a soothing alternative for children, who are often unable to handle more powerful migraine medications. However, I am leery of giving children any questionable medications—and remember, these folk remedies are medicines. Before trying any treatment, see your pediatrician or your child's neurologist. And if you do get the nod from your doctor, keep in mind that, as with drug treatments, children should get only child-sized doses. For most folk remedies, very young migraineurs should be given just one quarter of the amount taken by an adult. Children older than five may be gradually introduced to half the adult dose. Only after age twelve can the dose begin to be raised to the full amount. A little honey or juice in teas might help this medicine go down.

Are there any herbs to avoid if you're a migraineur?

Few herbs are harmful to migraineurs as a group, but some of them impact on other conditions a sufferer may have. For instance, people who have problems with blood clotting should probably avoid feverfew, which may slow clotting in some users. Some herbs, like meadowsweet, vervain, lemon balm, and feverfew, contain tannins, which impede the breakdown of proteins if used over long periods. You may get an allergic reaction to an herbal remedy, although that's not too common. In some cases, an herbal medication may contain an element that you're already getting through prescription medication, and it may cause an overdose. Women who are pregnant should stay away from folk remedies until they've checked with their doctors; after all, these remedies are medicines, too. Read more about any herb you're considering, and ask your doctor about its impact on your other medications or conditions.

What is a homeopathic remedy?

Many people use the word homeopathy to mean folk remedies, herbal treatments, and vitamin regimens. But homeopathy actually refers to a system of medicine developed a hundred years ago by a German doctor. It is based on the belief that herbs, minerals, and other substances that produce symptoms similar to those of a disease or ailment can be used in minute amounts to stimulate a person's natural defenses. This science is still controversial with many physicians, like myself, who practice allopathy, which is sometimes called conventional or traditional medicine—even though it's what you probably think of as modern medicine. More and more doctors, however, recognize the value of balancing the latest innovations with traditional folk remedies, which are often based on sound common sense. A few of those remedies are homeopathic.

Why am I hearing so much about holistic medicine when it comes to migraine treatment?

Holistic medicine refers to the treatment of the whole patient—body, mind, and lifestyle—not simply one symptom or disorder that person is experiencing. It operates on the understanding that a disorder can affect every aspect of a person's body and life. That's no revelation to migraineurs! You can see that a holistic approach is a natural one for migraine sufferers, many of whom are already practicing it unconsciously in their efforts to combine trigger maintainance, stress reduction, and pharmacological treatments. In order for a holistic approach to really work on migraine, all the people involved in your treatment need to work in concert with you *and* each other. That includes physicians, dietitians, physical therapists, psychologists, and any other professional involved in your care.

I've heard that belladonna helps, but isn't it poisonous?

Belladonna is one of the treatments used under the homeopathic umbrella. This is a very dicey treatment, with benefits that aren't supported by research. Since belladonna is a powerful poison when taken in the wrong amount, it is not a treatment you want to try on your own. Few doctors are likely to "prescribe" this particular treatment, so use caution if it's recommended for your migraine attacks. However, many doctors recommend Bellergal-S, a prescription drug that includes belladonna as one of its ingredients.

I saw incense labeled as a stress reliever. Can it help?

The use of incense is still a debatable form of treatment. Some patients say they have gotten relief from using this and other forms of aromatherapy. Certainly it can't hurt to use incense, unless scents are a trigger for you. The varieties reported to work on headache pain vary from manufacturer to manufacturer, so ask at the shops where you find incense. Some are labeled as stress or tension relievers, rather than migraine cures, and that is perhaps the secret of their success: They induce a state of peacefulness that helps alleviate the pain of an attack.

Will garlic pills fight my migraine?

No studies exist to support the effects of garlic on migraine. Anecdotal accounts say it prevents attacks by regulating fat in the bloodstream and improving blood flow. If this is eventually proven, be aware that adding garlic to your cooking won't help. Cloves should be eaten raw for the full effect. Luckily, capsule forms of garlic are available now with none of the malodorous side effects of the raw plant.

Will massage pressure on my scalp help relieve the pain or just make it worse?

Scalp massage often helps relieve headache pain. This may be due to the application of pressure on dilated blood vessels under the scalp or just the relaxation induced by the soothing movements. As long as you don't bear down too firmly, pressure is harmless. Many patients report getting relief by simply pressing down with their fingertips and moving their scalps back and forth gently. Others use a pattern of pressure points. Starting high on your forehead, centered above your nose at the hairline, press your thumb or two fingers down for a moment. Slowly work your way up the center of your skull, over your head, and down to the base of your skull, by one-inch measures. Then start at the top of your head and work your way down to one ear. Repeat on the other side. Even though it may act as a trigger for some sufferers, wearing a hat or headband can help once a headache arrives. You may have to keep it on until the attack runs its course, because, as with other applied-pressure techniques, the pain usually comes back when pressure is removed.

Which type of massage works best for migraine?

All kinds of massage have been reported to be effective in relieving headache pain or reducing the levels of stress that may trigger an attack. Some people have managed to head off an attack if they get a massage at the first hint of a migraine. The downside is that its effects are often as fleeting as the massage itself—once the soothing hands are taken away, the pain floods back. Still, it's worth it for those few minutes of relief and relaxation. For the best results you should visit a trained massage therapist. Massage that focuses on the head and neck seems to help migraine just as much as whole-body massage, but see which works for you. See if your physician will refer you to a massage therapist; virtually every medical insurance company requires a referral before they'll pay for this type of treatment.

I can't afford a professional massage. What can I do at home?

You can perform some massage moves yourself, like circular motions with fingertips pressed against your temples.

Or, to relieve headache pain centered over the sinus area, start with two fingers of each hand positioned between your brows. Pull back along the top of your eyebrows back to your temples. Another move to try is sweeping down and out across your cheeks from the bridge of your nose, using all your fingertips. Other moves are easier for a partner to perform. You may want to lie down with your partner seated behind your head, or you can sit, with your partner standing behind you. The massage begins with fingers pressed down on your shoulders and drawn up along the sides of the neck to just behind the ear. Other movements start at the temples and pull up and back into the hairline above the ears. Others work the area of your neck on either side of the spine.

Someone told me about some magical pressure point on your hand that can relieve headache pain. Where is that?

Many migraineurs report quick, if temporary, relief when they apply pressure to the fleshy area between the thumb and forefinger. Stop if pressure becomes painful. Pregnant women are usually warned against using this and other pressure points that target organs.

When should someone see a chiropractor?

Chiropractic treatments refer to the manipulation of the head, neck, and back through a series of twisting movements called "adjustments." It is yet another controversial treatment. Some people claim that these adjustments relieve the muscle tensions that can trigger a migraine. But a careless adjustment of the head or neck can put pressure on one of the many blood vessels found there, causing a stroke. Although such an occurrence is rare; because of the potential danger involved, the benefits of chiropractic treatment should be carefully considered and discussed with your doctor. Furthermore, chiropractic adjustments aren't always covered by insurance companies.

What about acupuncture as a treatment?

While it's true that some people report a benefit from acupuncture, the number of patients that report lasting benefits is relatively low. The traditional thought behind acupuncture is that it redirects the flow of energy known as the life force—*chi* or *chi'i*—through one of twelve major meridians (imaginary lines on the body's surface) and 365 points around your body. The scientific interpretation is that the pinpoint pressure of the needles causes your body to release endorphins, the substance so effective in pain relief. If this is an avenue you feel you want to try, ask your doctor for a referral to a reputable acupuncturist.

How painful is acupuncture—truly?

If acupuncture is done correctly, it's not painful, although many people find it a little uncomfortable, especially at first. The sensation is an odd one, and some people never get used to it. The most you should feel is a tingling or a slight, focused ache. If the needles cause you to bleed, they are not being applied correctly! It is essential that needles be disposed of or sterilized after each use, so ask what happens to the needles used in your sessions. Pain comes only with a misplaced needle, which can also be dangerous. However, if your therapist is well trained, the pain will be minimal.

What other forms of physical therapy should I try?

Even though they were annoying, all those lectures to "Sit up straight!" and "Bend with your knees" really were for your own good. Good posture is one very basic form of physical therapy that can have a significant effect. Pay attention to how you sit, stand, walk, and pick up heavy loads. If your job causes you to gradually slump into a hunched position over a computer or phone, straighten your back, drawing yourself upward from the hips. Press your shoulders back; hold your stomach in. Position your feet flat on the floor. If you're sitting still for long periods, deliberately relax your muscles with a good stretch at frequent intervals. While standing, shift your weight from one foot to the other, with legs shoulder-width apart. Avoid sudden moves from a seated or lying position: Roll out of bed and swing in and out of a car with your legs together, instead of twisting your upper body to one side. Attention to posture will help prevent exertion migraine attacks and those triggered by tense muscles.

What kind of exercise routine should I have as a migraineur?

Keeping your body healthy in general can help you battle the effects of a migraine attack. Exercise can also be a stress-buster, redirecting the adrenaline surge you get in tense situations. So establish a routine you perform regularly when pain-free. A combination of exercises gets the best results for a migraineur. Balance your cardiovascular workouts, which raise your heart rate, with toning or resistance exercises, such as free-weight training, crunches, and stretches. Cardiovascular exercises such as running, biking, stair climbing, rowing, and aerobics promote more efficient blood flow. This can help reduce the number and severity of your headaches. Toning exercises improve overall health and posture. Stretching helps with relaxation and aids circulation, so incorporate gentle head rotations, shoulder rolls, arm swings, huglike squeezes, front and side bends and twists—as well as others recommended by your doctor or therapist—into every workout session.

What should I do if exercise makes my migraine worse?

I frequently hear patients report exercise as a trigger, especially those who are runners. Fortunately for them, certain drugs can be taken prior to exercise to prevent the migraine from taking hold. Indomethacin is one of the drugs used to treat these exertional headaches; it's also effective against headaches which occur with orgasm. Even if exertion is one of your triggers and there are reasons not to use this drug therapy, don't cut exercise out of your life: there are too many other health benefits to consider. Instead, extend your warmup period, adding more slow stretches. That can halt the triggering effect. Slowly build up the length and difficulty of your basic exercises. You'll gradually expand your limits until you can do a complete routine without an attack. Eat a light snack soon after you exercise, and drink plenty of water during your routine. Hunger or dehydration might be your trigger, not exercise. But remember, when a headache does arrive, exercise can be your worst enemy. If *any* kind of movement makes your head throb—stop moving!

What is biofeedback anyway?

Biofeedback is a technique that enables patients to control some of their bodies' hidden mechanisms. It's centered around the belief that when you know exactly how the body performs a certain function, you can manipulate that action. Biofeedback helps migraineurs control a fairly universal symptom of an attack: cold hands and feet. What's amazing is that when the temperature of those extremities is returned to normal, other symptoms of migraine fade or disappear, too—such as headache pain. The key is visualizing the change and then willing it to happen. So, once you understand precisely how blood flows to your fingertips and feet, you can visualize the blood pumping through those arteries and veins, warming your feet and hands. You can picture your skin temperature rising. Through biofeedback, you train yourself to create these changes in your body any time, any place.

What can I expect from a biofeedback session?

For biofeedback to work, you first have to be able to "visualize" what's happening inside your body during migraine and in the healthy periods between attacks. So a therapist needs to know how your particular migraine presents itself and how your body works overall. A first appointment is usually an in-depth question-and-answer session very similar to the ones you have with headache specialists, including questions about medical history, diet, stress triggers, and lifestyle. A headache diary is a typical next step in the process. You probably will not begin your biofeedback training until a second session. The delay is necessary and worthwhile, because you both need to understand how your particular body functions in order for the biofeedback to work. On that visit, you'll be shown the equipment, which may be one or more machines that register changes in your body. These may include a surface electromyogram, or EMG, which shows the results when you consciously tighten and release muscles. Contractions directly affect the flow of blood to muscles and skin. Other machines record your skin temperature and brain waves. You'll be taught how to watch the signals they produce. Throughout the training process, these signals from the machines—beeps, hums, or flashing lights—

will tell you when temperature is rising or falling. You'll learn how to change the temperature levels through breathing exercises and relaxed concentration.

Is biofeedback training difficult to learn or painful?

This procedure is painless, but some people find that the pressure of responding to the signals is too stressful. For them biofeedback doesn't work because they can't relax to the point where they can make use of the training. For many patients, however, the training sessions become routine, and after about six sessions, you're able to produce the same results on your own, wherever you happen to be. Once training sessions are over, you control this therapy.

Can I teach myself biofeedback?

Some people try to teach themselves biofeedback. Although they may get results similar to relaxation techniques, they're not getting the maximum benefits of biofeedback. For that, you need to be trained by a professional. Despite its stress-reducing benefits, biofeedback is not considered a relaxation technique but a physiological one that uses special equipment. The trick is to find a good biofeedback therapist. Unlike medical doctors, therapists aren't regulated by rigidly controlled standards. So be sure to check into the background of the therapist you choose. Look for conventional medical or psychology training, and ask questions about the newer drug treatments for headache pain to see if your practitioner is up to date on the latest science behind migraine.

Does biofeedback really work on migraines?

Many patients have an excellent response to biofeedback. Children are the most likely to pick up on this technique and use it effectively if they think it's a game. But even the oldest patients can learn it. Some patients use biofeedback every day as a preventive therapy; others slip into a session only when the first migraine indicator appears. Both techniques seem to work; use the one that's best for you. The first studies documenting biofeedback's effectiveness against migraine were presented over twenty years ago in a study at the Meninger Clinic in Kansas. Since then, countless articles have documented results from other research. The anecdotal

evidence is overwhelming as well; many migraineurs tell stories about how it's worked for them. Perhaps because it is a
product of modern medicine—even though it has ancient origins—doctors tend to find it easier than other alternatives to
accept and are more likely to offer referrals covered by insurance for this alternative than for others. Biofeedback is
one of the nondrug alternatives I recommend to many of my
patients.

What role can meditation play in relieving my pain?

Anything that helps you manage stress and take control
over your body can help you in the treatment of migraine,
and meditation can accomplish both. Studies show that
through meditation you can learn to control breathing, blood
pressure, and heart rate. Other benefits include the treatment
of insomnia and headache pain reduction. For some people,
meditation may mean a few moments of quiet relaxation
spent mentally replaying scenes that bring feelings of seren-
ity. Mantras are code words chanted repeatedly to induce an
almost trancelike state; they're used in another form of meditation known as transcendental meditation, or TM. In traditional TM, you must be given a unique mantra, but many
Westerners use the generic Chinese "om," meaning whole.
It is repeated over and over in a low monotonous tone, drawing out both the *o* and the *m* sounds. You might find it helps
to perform a more modern version of this ancient Zen technique, repeating a simple sentence, such as "I deserve to feel
better," called an affirmation. This sentence can change from
day to day to reflect some positive, esteem-building situation
in your life, such as "I accomplished something today" or
"I am in control." Some people just hum. Others pray. Not
everyone can use meditation methods effectively, however,
so don't be disappointed if you don't get dramatic results or
if it takes time to see a change. If meditation simply helps
you feel more relaxed, it's still worth the effort.

What are some relaxation techniques I can use on my migraine?

The most effective relaxation techniques are the ones that
help you control your breathing. Deep breathing is a simple
technique anyone can master with practice. Concentrate on

slow, deep breaths: Inhale through your nose and exhale through your mouth in a steady and gentle manner. Begin each breath from your diaphragm. Hold your hand against your stomach and feel the inhalation start from there, instead of in your chest, and move up your body. Don't stop after a few breaths; keep the pattern going until you fall into an instinctive rhythm. Eventually, you'll drift off into a trance-like state in which your whole body releases tension. Try it lying down.

More sophisticated techniques like progressive muscle relaxation use deep breathing as one element of an even more complete relaxation. Many people do some form of this technique already, by concentrating on the relaxation of tense muscles. Progressive muscle relaxation works the same way but is a bit more systematic. You begin at your feet, deliberately releasing tension in that one spot. How can you relax a muscle at will? First, tighten it. The act of contracting the muscle is conscious, so relaxing it becomes conscious, too. After clenching each set of muscles for a few seconds, release them, focusing on one muscle group at a time: first your toes, then up along your legs, stomach, chest, hands, and arms. Now focus on your face and head. Frown, puckering up your whole face, then release those facial muscles. Raise your eyebrows as high as they'll go, then relax your forehead and scalp. During this step-by-step process, you should be taking long, slow breaths. At first, it may seem as though this is too much to think about all at once, but by the time you get to your face, you may find yourself performing the clench-release action without thinking too much about it, and the tension will have left your whole body.

What about yoga?

Yoga is yet another form of relaxation. It also centers around the control of your breathing and relaxation, through gentle, highly controlled stretches, postures, and movements. Although many books and videos teach yoga, it's best to learn from a teacher who can structure your yoga session around the needs of a migraine patient, since this technique is used to help a variety of conditions.

I can't concentrate on relaxing my muscles once pain hits. Is there a quicker relaxation technique?

If you have trouble focusing on muscle groups, try a technique called visualization or guided imagery. One day when you're not having an attack, think of a place or picture that has pleasant, soothing associations: lazily swaying in a hammock beside a Caribbean sea; clipping flowers in a shaded garden; or reading a bedtime story with your children. Take some time to picture that location or scene in detail. Listen to music that enhances that calming sensation. Then, when an attack strikes, find a quiet place where you can spend some minutes revisiting that setting. With practice, you should be able to slide right into the setting, pushing pain aside. Other people visualize the pain lifting from their heads as if it were a cloud or solid mass. They push the pain away from them and visualize themselves as being pain-free. Some imagine a color they find particularly serene, then imagine it filling them with every inhalation. Find an image that works for you. Relaxation techniques like these can be mastered on your own, but if you're having trouble or think you can get even better results, a psychologist should be able to help you discover your most effective and personalized images.

Is autogenic training the same as biofeedback?

Autogenic training is a term used to describe a technique similar to self-hypnosis. It literally means "self-born or self-produced." Psychologists are usually the best source for training in this technique. Basically, through autogenic training you learn to create special effects within your own body, without the use of any outside agent. Biofeedback is similar, but autogenic training doesn't involve the use of equipment to cue your responses. Instead, you learn a series of phrases, such as "My leg feels heavy and warm." You begin by simply saying the words. With practice, the power of suggestion makes those words become reality. You'll begin to relax and generate a response to match each phrase as you think it. Because it doesn't use beeping machines and sensors, autogenic training is a good option for people who get stressed out from the pressures of biofeedback or progressive relaxation. Not everyone can learn autogenics, but it can be an effective treatment for others.

If you can treat a headache with biofeedback and relaxation, is it really a migraine?

If it matches the criteria for migraine and if your history supports that diagnosis, then it's a migraine. If biofeedback and relaxation techniques help you control it, there's no reason to change that diagnosis; just reason to celebrate.

How can hypnosis help?

Hypnosis is not a widely accepted form of treatment or one I generally recommend; many doctors hesitate to suggest it because it doesn't seem to have any kind of lasting effect on migraine pain. On the other hand, some patients might find it helpful for dealing with stress, and it has been effective in that capacity. However, be wary of hypnotherapists who say they can make headache pain go away at the mention of some planted code word, or who urge you to come back for repeated sessions when initial visits aren't successful. Your therapist should explain that hypnosis helps you by distracting your attention away from headache pain, and preparing you for relaxation and body-controlling techniques. Some relaxation techniques, such as visualization, act as forms of self-hypnosis. These mild forms of hypnosis are at the very least harmless, and some sufferers report that it works for them. Look for hypnotherapists who are also licensed physicians, psychologists, or psychotherapists.

What about oxygen? Will it help my migraines?

Breathing pure oxygen has proven very effective in the treatment of cluster headache, but it appears to be virtually useless against migraine. Patients can order tanks and oxygen through surgical supply houses, keeping the tank near the bedside for quick treatment of the typical predawn attacks of cluster. Oxygen treatment needs to be administered under the care of a doctor, however, so don't experiment with it without professional help.

What are trigger point injections?

Sometimes called TPT, for trigger point therapy, this treatment is precisely what it sounds like: A doctor injects a needle into specific sites along your neck and shoulders, where the tense muscles triggering headache pain are usually located. A general practitioner, neurologist, or anesthesiologist can perform this therapy. This is a relatively new practice so few studies exist to support its efficiency against migraine. There isn't much anecdotal evidence either, since shots of any kind aren't the most popular treatments. It doesn't help that trigger point injections are expensive and patients usually need to have repeated applications of TPT before showing signs of improvement.

Which vitamins and minerals should I be taking?

Once again, this varies from patient to patient. You take vitamin supplements to replace those you lack, so check with a doctor to see if you have any vitamin deficiencies. In my experience, vitamin supplements don't offer chronic sufferers much help; they're more effective for the maintenance of general well-being. However, some are recommended by doctors for migraineurs, to combat the losses that result from drug and other treatments. These include vitamins E, C, and some B complex vitamins. Studies suggest that vitamin C assists the effects of aspirin. The popularity of magnesium supplements seems to be increasing. Magnesium is commonly sold as Epsom salts, in crystal or powder form. Other minerals that might be recommended include boron, chrominum picolinate, copper, potassium, and zinc. The amount of a vitamin or mineral taken may be highly individual so be sure to ask what the right amount is for you. Some must be taken with meals or at other specific times; find out more details about any supplements your doctor suggests.

Which vitamins and minerals should I avoid?

Large amounts of vitamins A and D can actually cause headaches, as a result of tissue damage caused by an excess of these vitamins. They can also damage the kidney when taken in high doses, which leads to an increase of blood calcium, another headache trigger. Liver has high levels of vitamin A, so watch the amount you eat.

A woman tried to sell me migraine-fighting magnets in the lobby of my doctor's building. Should I have bought one?

Migraine pain may feel like a nail being driven through your head, but no magnet is going to draw it out. Magnets are one of the quack remedies sometimes pedaled to migraineurs. Some sufferers experience pain so excruciating that anything sounds good. This is one method that has no validity, however, so steer clear. Be wary of any "cure" being sold through such casual contact. And let your doctor know that his lobby is being used for the sale of snake oil.

What is TENS?

TENS is the acronym for transcutaneous electrical nerve stimulation. That's a complicated label for what is really focused electrical shocks to areas of the body feeling pain. It may sound like something from a science-fiction or prison-torture movie, but some patients have reported getting relief from this treatment. The benefits, if any, are temporary, and the treatment can only be used when an attack is in progress. Since sufferers must schedule appointments with a physical therapist for a TENS treatment, timing can be tricky. Like many other physicians, I'm doubtful about the use of TENS on migraine pain and will hold out for further studies before recommending this treatment to my patients.

Can seasickness wristbands alleviate the nausea of my migraines?

Limited success has been reported with these wristbands for helping with the nausea that accompanies most migraine attacks. However, the same mixed response is also the case when the wristbands are used for their original purpose. The bands are relatively inexpensive and have no side effects, so migraineurs who are aware of a motion-sickness trigger to their migraine should try this method if they're going on a trip, whether on land or sea.

Is it wishful thinking that sex helps alleviate an attack?

Many migraineurs report that sex can lessen the pain of the attack. Others experience the relatively rare case of exertional headache, which may be triggered by the act. This is one of those "treatments" that's highly individual. If it works for you, and your partner is willing to join in with your therapy, by all means continue this form of treatment!

Do diving chambers really work?

Hyperbaric oxygen, or diving, chambers work only on cluster headache, not migraine. They're not found in every hospital, but if you can get access to one, be prepared to pay through the nose. It's an expensive process and must be performed by hospital staff. This isn't a very practical option for most patients.

My friend says throwing up helps ease the pain. Is it wise to do this on purpose?

Sometimes being sick is not an option. But it's true many migraineurs report feeling better after throwing up, and some induce vomiting because they know the pain will stop afterward. Of course, that may occur only because vomiting is a signal of the end-cyle of your unique migraine attack. Talk to your doctor before making a practice of induced vomiting. Concerns naturally arise when the behavior becomes addictive, if your body has trouble replacing lost fluids and nutrients, or if controlled vomiting for the sake of migraine masks a problem with dieting and self-image, such as anorexia. You may not be able to see these patterns yourself. For those sufferers on the other end of the spectrum—the ones who find the vomiting the worst part of the attack—Imitrex (sumatriptan) has been found to relieve that symptom, as well as persistent nausea.

Sometimes hyperventilating works for me. Is it safe?

Breathing into a paper bag as soon as you spot the symptoms of aura may help by briefly increasing your levels of carbon dioxide. Don't ever cover your whole head, however, and don't use the paper-bag technique once the headache arrives—it will just make it worse at that stage.

Are there any quick fixes?

You know there's no real fix, but there are some quick and easy tips that migraineurs pass along for managing migraine attacks. Here are some of the most common: Drink lots and lots of water. Get a larger computer monitor with a higher refresh rate (the higher the refresh rate, the easier on your eyes—and on your headache) or add an antiglare screen to your computer. Snack frequently on healthy foods, especially those popular with athletes, such as high-fiber bars, apple juice, and handfuls of grain cereal. Switch between reading glasses and other lenses instead of using bifocals that make you tip your head back. Don't tilt your head back when shaving under your chin. Drive with the steering wheel closer to your body, so you don't slump. Switch from sports like football, rowing, and snowmobiling—sports with movements that seem to trigger headache—to cycling, tennis, racquetball, volleyball, and swimming. Jump in a shower that's as hot or cold as you can handle, or alternate back and forth between temperatures (this hot and cold therapy is called *diathermy*). Apply hot or cold compresses to the neck and head, especially the spot against the base of the skull. Take a warm bath. Sleep on your back with a pillow under your knees. If you can't get used to that position, cut down on body stress by sliding the pillow between your knees if you're a side sleeper or under your hips if you sleep on your stomach. Develop strategies for defusing your own stress triggers by first identifying what pushes you over the edge: Are you stretching yourself too thin, rushing from one thing to the next? Routinely carry a datebook and be firm about leaving an hour between every appointment. Do you begin to steam when waiting for friends who are always late? Show up late yourself, or bring along a crossword puzzle or Walkman to distract you from the minutes that are ticking by. If you're getting tense rushing to make a meeting, use deep-breathing techniques as you run. Use your deep breathing, too, whenever you need to catch up on lost sleep; in a pinch a few minutes of slow breathing can replace an afternoon nap. Integrate these and other alternatives with your traditional treatments. You're sure to find something in the wide range of nondrug alternatives that can alleviate some of the symptoms of migraine and help you feel more in control of yourself and your headaches.

TEN

Living with Migraine

CASE STUDY

Anita looked like a shadow when she first visited the clinic. Years of pain seemed to have worn her down to a thread. I got her started on biofeedback and Imitrex, which together took care of the worst of the pain, but that didn't solve the whole problem. It became clear that Anita didn't have much of a support network. As much as they loved her, Anita's family couldn't seem to understand what she was going through. She felt guilty complaining to them. Anita didn't have many close friends; she had always focused on her family, work, and migraine. I suggested she join a support group, but Anita offered a handful of excuses: she didn't have time; it was too inconvenient to travel; she was sure it wouldn't help. I suspected the real reason was shyness, and she admitted to feeling uncomfortable facing strangers. Anita was interested in one-to-one counseling but worried about being able to afford it with her less-than-generous health plan.

As I struggled to find ways to aid Anita with the emotional toll of migraine, she finally found a solution herself from a surprising source. Anita often cruised the Internet with her children. They created a home page with a section devoted to migraine. Soon, e-mail flooded in from sufferers all over the country, sharing their stories about migraine, offering advice, and asking questions about what worked for her. "Suddenly, I wasn't alone anymore," she told me. "People

*who didn't even know me cared about how I was doing. And
I realized I didn't have it nearly as bad as some others. The
whole thing was like a revelation.''*

The semianonymous support encouraged her to overcome
her shyness and find a local support group. Meetings with
other sufferers gave her a chance to sound off, and it helped
her family understand the disorder when she brought them
along to a meeting. In addition, working on the home page
together with her children made them more interested in migraine. Anita had an appointment recently and she showed
up a different person than the one who came to the clinic
two years ago. She has learned to live with migraine.

Because there is no cure for migraine, the key to living
with it revolves around control. As a migraineur, you have
to adopt a strategy that may seem contradictory at first: Battle
the disorder relentlessly and accept it, too.

For the battle against migraine, commit yourself to the
search for a treatment that will eliminate your attacks. The
weapons are out there somewhere. In the meantime, organize
your life so migraine is least disruptive. And if a headache
overwhelms you at times, that doesn't mean you've done
anything wrong. It's simply the nature of the beast. Taming
migraine isn't easy and there may be times when it takes a
savage bite. Accept it, and remember that every treatment
attempted is taking you one step closer to the solution that
works for you.

Begin living with migraine by creating a treatment team
of patient, doctor, family, co-workers, and friends. You're
the captain of that team, the one who will shape the actions
of all the others and take the lead in the battle against pain.
So if you say, ''It's okay, I can handle it,'' don't be surprised
when everyone believes you. That's the first lesson of living
with migraine: Honesty is a necessity. The second lesson:
Ask for help. Let your team know what they are doing to
make your migraine worse or better.

Be aware of what you do as well. The choices you make
every day will affect your migraine. Look carefully at yourself and your lifestyle, and be aware of the daily decisions
you're making and how they'll impact on headache pain. If
it's not a positive impact, change your behavior.

Start by paying attention to your body's natural rhythms and needs. If you feel tired and groggy in the late afternoon, remember that there's a reason why people take breaks. Plan less strenuous activities around your low points, and you'll have fewer headaches. Pace your activities to accommodate daily, weekly, and monthly cycles, and avoid booking activities for every night of the week. If you rely on your datebook, schedule some time to just relax and unwind. Prime your body to fight migraine through exercise and a nutritional, trigger-free diet.

If any of that seems like a waste of time, think of how many hours you're losing to migraine pain each week or month right now. Then make a few of the changes outlined in this chapter. Log how much time is spent in relaxation techniques, exercise, monitoring meals, or taking periodic stretching breaks at work. Are you really losing any time? Or does an hour's worth of daily maintenance save you a lost day or more each week?

Making changes that affect every aspect of your life—adapting work habits and environments, scheduling family meetings, being vigilant about exercise and menu planning—may seem inconvenient, time consuming, or just plain frustrating at first, but in the long run it's worth it. When you make the commitment to follow through on your treatment, the payoff is tremendous—no more migraine attacks! In the meantime, if you still get a headache, wait it out as you've done before. The pain will end, and someday soon you'll find a way to eliminate migraine once and for all, instead of finding ways to live with it.

My whole life centers on migraine. It's all I ever think about, even when I'm not having an attack. Is that normal?

When suffering with a chronic disorder like migraine, it's certainly normal to sometimes fixate on your condition, especially in the period surrounding an attack or in the course of developing a treatment plan. It's not unusual for people who suffer from chronic pain to become downright obsessive about their attacks. But just because it's normal doesn't mean it's healthy behavior. If you are spending all your migraine-free moments worrying about when your next attack will arrive, you are wasting your time.

There is one benefit to experiencing the pain of migraine, and that is truly appreciating what it is to be pain-free. A migraineur can revel in good health with an appreciation that nonsufferers will never know. So, when you have a pain-free day, simply enjoy it, without thinking about when another attack may arrive. Feeling positive isn't just a cliche when it comes to migraine, it's a treatment. Positive feelings have been shown to reduce stress, so by simply enjoying a pain-free day you may prevent an attack.

If thoughts of migraine are becoming obsessive, though, try scheduling specific times in which you can focus on the disorder: regular doctor visits, a five-minute daily entry in a headache diary, or sessions with support groups. Then, when the disorder begins to overwhelm your life, you can tell yourself, "Well, I'll have plenty of time to think about this on Friday, when I'm with my group." Sometimes knowing you'll have an opportunity to deal with your issues will enable you to "let go" at other times. If scheduled sessions to talk it out aren't feasible, try practicing the relaxation and visualization techniques outlined in Chapter 9, and learn to channel your thoughts into more positive, constructive directions. If you're still having trouble, get a referral to a therapist; together you'll discover other ways to conquer your obsession with your migraine disorder.

These attacks are happening to me, but how much are they affecting my family?

You won't know until you ask. Your migraine attacks may affect your family quite a bit, more or less than you're imagining. It all depends, of course, on how your family interacts, the kinds of activities you do together, your role in the household, and just how crippling your attacks can be. So, ask.

How can I ask my family to do things for me when I'm feeling sick all the time?

You can ask, and they can do. You undoubtedly do things for your family all the time, without questioning it. It is only fair and right that they should help out when help is needed. Ten to one, you're the only one who really thinks you're asking too much. However, if you're worried about burdening them too much or too often, talk to your family and see if they share this concern, and together work out ways to balance any unfair workload. Balance requests for help with special times and privileges that acknowledge the extra level of responsibility. Set aside time when you're feeling well to really focus on your family, even if it's one member at a time, doing something special for or with each one as a way of thanking them for the extra effort.

I feel guilty that my family has to put up with this. They seem so frustrated. How can I help them deal with it?

Much of the frustration your family expresses may simply be the result of feeling helpless. If you let them know what they can do to make things better, it will help them cope and at the same time provide you with the help you need to manage the pain. Involve family members in some of the decisions that revolve around migraine: planning family events that might be affected, eliminating triggers from the home, figuring out how to handle family routines when an attack disables you. Explore how they feel, what makes them worried, angry, or upset. You might start discussions by asking "How do you feel when . . ." and "What are some things *you* think will help?" Talking may not come easily to some families, but it's essential to ease the tensions you all may feel. If family members feel they can't openly discuss issues like these, encourage them to vent to others—a trusted friend or relative—who can act as an intermediary. If the rest of your family is involved in decisions, they're less likely to lash out later when attacks disrupt plans. But don't be surprised if they do! You may need to schedule a few family meetings to review some choices you've made together. One other thing to think about is helping yourself deal with the guilt. Perhaps the burden on your family isn't as great as the one you're placing on yourself. If guilty feelings begin to overwhelm you, a counselor should be able to find more ways for you to help yourself and your family cope with migraine.

My family isn't being very supportive. What can I do?

Be willing to compromise. If a family member's habits, such as smoking or playing loud music, contribute to your attacks, define limits for *both* of you: where and when he or she is allowed to indulge this habit and what you'll do on your part to avoid the triggering factor. Understand that it's natural for families to occasionally feel angry, disappointed, resentful, jealous of the attention, even guilty of being healthy—just as it's normal for you to sometimes feel left out, sorry for yourself, guilty, frustrated, and resentful of anyone who doesn't have the pain. Talk about it. And if "occasionally" is becoming "all the time," get help from other sources, such as support groups or family counseling.

How can I make my little ones understand why I'm acting so tired and mean?

Even very little children understand the concept of "boo-boos." If you tell them the boo-boo is inside your head and that they must be very, very quiet or your head will hurt, they can understand that. Some sufferers have suggested the trick of putting an adhesive bandage on your forehead when you're having an attack, as a visual reminder to children that your head doesn't feel very good. Set some ground rules for what happens at times when your head hurts: where children can play and what toys are good for quiet time. Explain how Mommy or Daddy might behave; that you might be cranky— but do it first on a day when you're pain-free. Remind them what to do at regular intervals. That way you'll all be ready on days when an attack hits.

When I'm having an attack, the last thing I want to do is sit around explaining how bad it is, so what can I do?

Assign ratings to the different levels of pain you experience during attacks, describing what each level of pain feels like in the most precise terms you can find. Write them out for your family during a pain-free period and give a copy to each member. These ratings will let everyone know exactly how to "score" each attack and what your family can do to make you feel better. You might use the same ratings you develop with your doctor for your headache diary, or come up with definitions that are clearer to your children. For example, a level 1 headache might be described as: "I can handle conversation and participate in family activities, but

I may seem a little out of it and cranky, so please be patient and take things slow.'' A level 5 might then be listed as: ''Don't even *tiptoe* past the bedroom. My head is about to explode. Just play quietly in the basement until Daddy comes home and don't expect to see me for the next six hours.'' Then, when an attack strikes, all you'll need to do is whisper ''level 5'' as you make a beeline for your darkened bedroom. Everyone will know exactly what that means.

My companion doesn't understand the kind of agony I'm in. Short of banging my better half over the head to provide an idea of what the pain's like, what can I do to get some understanding?

Besides experience, education is the best cure for ignorance. Find the description of pain that finally ''clicks.'' If language doesn't work, draw pictures. Migraineurs have created some pretty compelling portraits of the pain they feel. Invite companions to read the literature you've collected. Introduce them to the Internet to experience the countless case histories posted there. Visit support groups to meet other families of sufferers. Ask *them* what would help them understand.

How can I explain why I act so different around the time of an attack—depressed, edgy, and angry?

It helps to explain in advance of an attack that your emotions can be as ragged as your pain, so companions are prepared when pain makes you say or do things that seem out of character, or just plain mean. Explain that the physical changes occurring in your brain have psychological effects, symptoms produced because the mechanics of migraine are affecting different centers in your brain, including those that control mood, emotional responses, and senses.

I'm giving this book to my companion, who gets migraines. What else can I do to help?

Simply by asking the question, you're indicating willingness to provide the best support you can give. It would be impossible not to be occasionally angered or disappointed, in fact, to experience a whole range of unpleasant emotions. It's how you manage your reactions to these feelings that can positively impact a loved one with migraine. Be flexible about changing plans. Express a willingness to learn more about headache. Encourage migraineurs in the sometimes tedious round of therapy experiments. Remind them to take their medication. Listen. Or creep away from the room quietly when nothing can help but darkness and silence. Just that may be enough.

Nothing worked for my mom—does that mean I'll be living with migraine pain the rest of my life, too?

You might have inherited a predisposition for migraine, but that doesn't mean you have the same type of headache as your parent, or that you're doomed to suffer if nothing worked for her. Your headaches may respond well to the very same treatments that did not succeed with her. Then again, there are many more treatment options today than in the past, so there are countless more alternatives for you to explore. Also, your mother may have adopted an attitude of silent suffering, or given up on finding relief if the first treatment didn't work, if she ever sought help for her headaches at all. You shouldn't feel obliged to continue that family tradition. There's no reason to believe that your headaches are untreatable just because a relative's were—just the opposite, in fact. You'd be a very rare case if you didn't find relief! Nowadays, the philosophy of "doomed to failure" is just an excuse not to try.

My treatment seems to be working for me, but my friend says the drug she's using is better. Should I switch?

If you're doing fine on your treatment, and your physician isn't concerned about your therapy, stick with it. Just because it doesn't work for another sufferer doesn't mean your treatment plan isn't effective; on the contrary, migraine's highly individual nature makes it unlikely that the exact same combination of factors will work for both you and your friend. By the same token, you shouldn't be discouraged when a treatment that's effective on others doesn't bring you any relief. Stick to what works for you.

How should I manage my diet with migraine?

Once you've identified your food triggers, the real challenge of learning to use this knowledge begins. Incorporating what you know about food triggers into a busy lifestyle is challenging, especially when you find yourself in a world of nonsufferers.

The best way to manage your diet is to know precisely what you're eating. That means knowing what's in the foods you purchase at the grocery store as well as in what you order at a restaurant. Read food labels. Ask about the ingredients in restaurant dishes. If you feel awkward or embarrassed about interrogating your waiter, think of yourself as coming across as a knowledgeable and discriminating consumer. In managing your migraine at home, be aware of how and when taking food affects your headache. For instance, morning headache sufferers sometimes get relief if they plan ahead by eating a high-protein snack or drinking a sweet drink at bedtime to prevent low morning blood sugar levels. If a headache still seems imminent in the morning, try sipping a cup of caffeinated coffee or tea as soon as you wake up. The diet that's recommended for general good health—cutting back on the sugar, salt, and fat—may eliminate diet-related triggers and have a beneficial effect on migraine.

Will changing my eating patterns during the day help my headache?

Sometimes it's not having enough food in your system, rather than eating the wrong kind, that brings on migraine. If hunger's your trigger, try eating between four to six small meals spread evenly throughout the day. Keep these meals as nutritionally balanced as a larger meal, though; don't rely on fatty, high-calorie snack foods to bridge the gaps. Eat when you're hungry and stop when you're full, because overeating can be a trigger, too. Another way to make living with migraine easier is to eat the same kind of foods on weekends as during the week, and in similar time patterns. Sudden shifts may contribute to weekend headaches.

Will exercise just improve my quality of life or will it actually help fight migraine?

Improving your quality of life is reason enough to stick to an exercise routine, but, yes, exercise does seem to help some sufferers manage headache pain. Many report that a brisk walk, jog, or low-impact workout at the first sign of a headache has stopped the pain of an attack in its tracks. Most doctors recommend a minimum of three twenty- to sixty-minute sessions per week to maintain good health in general. That appears to be a good criterion for migraine sufferers as well.

In addition to its preventive benefits, exercise on a regular basis can help your body deal with headache pain more effectively, since any disorder is better fought by a healthy body. By exercising, you gain more control over your body and get a better idea of how it functions, both of which can help you use biofeedback more efficiently. You're less likely to give in to diet temptations and sabotage yourself by binging on chocolate or splurging on MSG-laden food, when you've already invested so much effort in yourself. Regular exercise promotes relaxation, too.

However, the best benefit of exercise is the self-esteem you get from the results, which triggers the release of endorphins. These mood-boosting chemicals assist in combating migraine pain, but good feelings about yourself may prevent some tension triggers from ever taking hold.

I'm a manager who needs to concentrate at work. What can I do to keep my focus during an attack?

Assuming that you haven't yet found the combination of drugs and other therapies that works for you, headache at work can be a big problem. But there are ways to deal with these attacks. First, though, ask yourself: Does the pressure to forge ahead regardless of the pain come from the work situation or from my own impossible standards? Sometimes migraineurs become obsessed with presenting an image of control, going beyond what's really necessary in order to compensate for their disorder.

When pain strikes next time, try to delegate some of the work that needs focused attention. Force yourself to let go of some control. Evaluate what really requires your personal attention and pass along the work that doesn't. Or save simple but necessary tasks for days when you've got pain. That's the time to tidy your office, weed out old files, or do other low-concentration tasks. Give yourself that time out. Pushing yourself through a high-focus job may just make the attack worse or last longer, which just ends up wasting more of your time.

If you must concentrate on work during an attack, take a break now and then to stretch and relax. Loosen tense muscles and rest strained eyes by relaxing for a few minutes. Try relaxation techniques such as deep breathing to focus your mind and alleviate the pain that's distracting you. Finally, recognize that there may be times when you're simply not able to concentrate on anything but the pain, no matter what you do. Accept it. Know your limits and respect them—that's an important part of controlling your migraine.

Should I tell my boss I get migraines?

The answer to this is different for every migraineur. For some, who are able to function normally during an attack, raising the subject with a boss seems irrelevant, even damaging. They believe that a boss might start looking for signs of problems that don't exist, or measure performance with a different yardstick. Even when headaches result in repeated absences, some migraineurs hide the disorder, choosing instead to invent a string of excuses. That may work for those whose migraine attacks are mild and easily disguised.

For others, the situation is not so easily kept under their hats. Being more open about their disorder may be the only option.

For others, revelation is a deliberate choice. Look at what you hope to gain by telling an employer, and see if it is worth the potential risks. If you do tell your boss, go armed with information. Have a plan ready, covering how you'll make up work and meet responsibilities. Talk about what the disorder is and how you're managing it. Don't look for pity or comfort; instead present your information as a series of facts and be ready with concrete assurances (it hasn't affected your productivity in the long run) and suggestions (replacing the fluorescent bulbs in my office with standard lamps will help). That's a much more effective strategy for getting results than asking for sympathy.

What can I do to reduce attacks at the office or cope with ones I get while I'm working?

Some steps you can take are simple and discreet things you can do yourself, such as adjusting the contrast and brightness of your computer monitor, buying shades for a sunlit window, bringing in lamps to help equalize light in your office, cutting down on fluorescent triggers, finding back supports for your office chair, quietly closing the door now and then for a stretch to release tension, speaking privately to cologne-wearing co-workers about scent triggers, wearing earplugs to cut down on noise triggers, keeping your own stock of decaffeinated drinks and nontrigger snacks, and plugging up air vents that blow on your neck. If you work long hours at the computer, set an alarm to remind you to take a break every forty-five minutes or so—do some neck stretches. If you're on the phone constantly, invest in a headset so you're not awkwardly cradling a phone between your ear and shoulder. Choose a chair that lets you sit up straight comfortably, supports your back, and allows you to rest your feet flat on the floor.

What if making my life easier makes my co-workers' lives harder?

Before you ask for major changes in the office, educate anyone who might be affected by adjustments you request. If they know how painful the attacks are, how easily they can be avoided, and how much more efficiently you'll be able to respond to their requests and support them, co-workers and bosses will be more amenable to changes in the office. Some of these changes may include switching offices with someone so you're no longer near a sunny window, covering the zigzag-patterned carpet with an inexpensive solid-color floor covering, putting a low-priced sofa in a room that can be your sanctuary if you need to lie down in a darkened room. If lying down quietly helps alleviate headaches, explain to others that while you'll be unavailable for an hour or so, lying down will prevent you from losing a whole day or more.

Living with office migraine works both ways, though, so be sure you make co-workers aware that you'll do your part: Develop strategies to make up for lost time. Plan ahead for emergencies by keeping others up to date on projects so your work is covered when you're absent. Arrange files and records in a neat and rational manner, as clearly labeled as possible, in case someone needs to access them when you're unavailable. You should be willing to bring work home or come in on weekends if you need to make up lost time.

I've taken all my sick days as a result of migraine attacks. What do I do now?

That's a good question for you to discuss with your boss or human resources department. If your migraine attacks are chronic and excruciating, you might qualify for disability. Familiarize yourself with your company's disability, leave of absence, and emergency leave policies. Find out the current status of the Americans with Disabilities Act; it grants you certain rights if you meet the criteria for disability. Perhaps you can work out an option to a standard work week, like "flex time," which allows you to arrive at work earlier or later in the day. Adjust the schedule around the hours you're most likely to experience migraine. Some flex-time plans allow you to work at home on sick days. Becoming a contract employee or working out a job-sharing arrangement, rather than remaining full time, can give you more flexibility, too, but it usually means a cut in pay or benefits. Bargain for benefits or options that seem most important, like medical insurance.

Clearly, how far a company is willing to go will be based on how much you can give them in return. Evaluate ways you can bring something special to the company—for instance, increased loyalty and commitment. Let them know you're willing to go the extra mile. Go to meetings prepared to persuade and inform, rather than in a combative or demanding frame of mind.

My migraines have gotten to the point where I can't work at my job anymore. What happens now?

If migraine prevents you from holding down your current job, even when undergoing treatment, find a job you can manage while dealing with migraine. That may seem like a ludicrous suggestion, one that ignores the financial and emotional toll of unemployment or a major job change, but it's simply a realistic assessment of your situation. If your migraine is disabling, changes must be made until you find a treatment that works for you. A major lifestyle change is certainly a frightening possibility, but it can also mean liberation from a no-win battle with pain. For some sufferers, leaving the nine-to-five work force has meant switching to a job in a more laid-back office or self-employment. Migraine was the force that led them in a new, more fulfilling direction and released them from tension triggers. It may do the same for you.

I flunked out of college because of my migraines. What can my daughter do to get by in that environment?

So many advances in the treatment of migraine have occurred in the last decade; your daughter's chances of success are probably greater than yours were at the time you were attending school. Nowadays, not only are more drugs that can help available but the philosophies of schools themselves have changed toward students with disabilities. Universities are more open to working out schedules to meet students' needs.

But your daughter can take proactive steps as well. Plan ahead to eliminate triggers in the school environment. Discuss this particular situation with your doctor to see what drugs work best in a school setting, and to discuss the possible side effects like drowsiness or confusion. Work with teachers and school authorities to create a schedule that accommodates periodic attacks. Create a network of classroom supporters who can help your daughter by sharing notes for missed classes and passing along assignment information.

How can changing my lifestyle affect my attacks?

It can have a huge impact. Behavior modification can control migraine just as drugs can. Maintaining a regular sleep pattern is one of the first lifestyle changes I recommend. On weekends, wake up at your normal weekday hour. Eat something, sip some tea, or use the bathroom, and *then* go back to bed to get some extra weekend hours of sleep. If you regularly awaken with headaches, you can prevent attacks by arranging your wake-up call or alarm for an hour or so earlier than you need it. Take your medicine and then sleep for another hour while it's taking effect.

Other lifestyle changes that are important, but may be more difficult, because of addictions, include quitting smoking and cutting back on alcohol. Keeping stricter control over your diet to eliminate triggers is another. It may seem like you're cutting all the enjoyment out of your life. But migraine attacks are probably cutting into your fun times more often than any of these lifestyle changes would. Seek help if you'd like to make changes but can't do it without support. Many people need professional counseling or other help to kick the habits that trigger migraine.

How will changing my drinking habits impact the frequency and severity of my headaches?

If you control your intake of alcohol, your headaches should lessen in number and severity. Drinking late at night, especially just before bed, may seem like the cure for your difficulty sleeping but it may actually be the cause of your insomnia. A nightcap has a boomerang effect. It makes you feel sleepy at first, but in a few hours the effects of the alcohol reverse, waking you and keeping you sleepless for hours. Try cutting back one glass a day, then more. You should notice a difference. Alcohol is one of the top five headache triggers, so it's likely that it's one of yours.

How do I deal with the anger when migraines prevent me from doing something I really want or need to do?

First, acknowledge that some headaches are bound to happen. Migraine attacks don't arrive at convenient moments—in fact, they often crop up at the least convenient times. Anxiety that you'll get a migraine may trigger attacks. If you find that migraine always interrupts important plans, don't just wait for the pain to hit. Be prepared. Talk to your doctor before a big event; perhaps you can explore preventive measures to take before the crucial time period. In the days before important events, try relaxation techniques. These techniques will also serve you well in dealing with any feelings of anger you have. Or make alternative plans—what will you and your friends or family do if you get an attack on the important day? Often, your anger stems from missing out on an event and feeling as if you've disappointed others. Sometimes knowing you have an escape route may relieve some of your tension. Plan activities with groups of friends, so that even if you can't make it, your friends' plans don't come to a standstill. Be aware of your own trigger events: If you often get headaches on weekends, plan more of your favorite activities during the week; if headaches are linked to your menstrual cycle, schedule them around it.

If migraine prevents participation in an activity, offer yourself a consolation prize, another favored thing or event to look forward to, once the pain is gone. Or pamper yourself to make up for the lost activity. Blaming yourself or your headache for bad timing just creates stress, which in turn prolongs the pain or brings on another migraine after an attack has passed.

If I could do just one thing on my own to improve my life with migraine, what would you suggest?

Finding and eliminating your triggers is perhaps the most important step to living with migraine, and it's one you can monitor yourself.

When should I just give up looking for relief?

Don't ever give up. The vast majority of sufferers get relief once they begin exploring ways to manage their migraine attacks. If you haven't found the right combination of pharmaceuticals, lifestyle changes, and alternative therapies yet, keep trying. You and your doctor may have to keep going back to the drawing board, which is tedious and frustrating, but your alternative is recurring pain. Keep looking for triggers that you may have missed during your initial observations, combinations of medication that work, or new drugs. Relief is out there—so why give up?

Modified* Headache Classification Chart

(includes broad diagnostic criteria for the primary disorders)

Primary headache—in order of frequency

- *Tension-type*: muscular contractions of the scalp, neck, and/or shoulders
- *Migraine*:
  - *Migraine without aura*: headache plus one of more generalized symptoms
    - *Abdominal migraine*: pain in stomach rather than head
    - *Benign exertional or orgasmic headache*: pain during sex or other activity
  - *Migraine with aura*: at least two attacks that feature aura
    - *Aphasic migraine*: ability to communicate though speech is affected
    - *Ataxic migraine*: balance and coordination are affected
    - *Aura without headache*: no head pain appears; other generalized symptoms
    - *Basilar artery migraine*: diminution of blood to the back of the brain causes dizziness, weakness
    - *Complicated migraine*: neurological symptoms persist after headache ends
      - *Familial hemiplegic migraine*: weakness of the extremities on same side as headache pain; solely in patients with family history of migraine
      - *Ophthalmoplegic migraine*: double vision
    - *Dysphrenic migraine*: symptoms and aura resemble psychiatric disturbances

---

*Some physicians recommend this modification to the standard chart to allow doctors to classify migraine more easily.

Source: *Handbook of Headache Disorders* by A. H. Elkind

- *Facial migraine*: intense pain in lower face and jaw
- *Hemisensory migraine*: tingling or prickling sensation in skin, face, lips, legs, and/or arms
- *Retinal migraine*: vision may dim or punch out; occasional permanent damage to vision
- *Cluster type*: attacks of short duration that occur in four- to six-week clusters

Secondary causes of headache

- *Traction causes*
  - Neoplasms
  - Hematomas
  - Hemorrhage
  - Thrombotic and ischemic disease
  - Expanding disease in the eyes, ears, nose, and throat structures
- *Inflammatory causes*
  - Giant cell arteritis with involvement of the cranial arterial structures
  - Collagen-vascular disorders
  - Infections of the meninges and surrounding structures of the head and neck
  - Brain abscess (may cause headache due to expansion as well)
  - Inflammatory disease of the venous system
  - Malignant hypertension with vascilitis
  - Inflammatory disease of the temporomandibular joint
  - Cranial neuralgias
- *Post-traumatic headache*
- *Miscellaneous*
  - Noncephalic infections
    - Influenza
    - Febrile disorders
  - Metabolic and endocrine disorders
    - Endocrine-pheochromocytoma
    - Carcinoid tumors
  - Chemical and pharmacological agents; mastocytosis

Headache Disability Rating

You can use this chart to figure out how to grade your migraine's severity. Multiply the rating for time lost from work by the rating for headache frequency, then match the number to one in the bottom section on the degree of disability.

Time Lost from Work or Routine Activity (Per Month)	Headache Rating
More than 72 hours lost	11
36–72 hours lost	10
16–36 hours lost	7
8–16 hours lost	5
2–8 hours lost	4
0–2 hours lost	3
Able to function during pain	2

Headache Frequency (Number of Headaches Per Month)	Headache Rating
10 or more headaches a month	11
7–9 headaches a month	9
4–6 headaches a month	7
2–3 headaches a month	4
1 headache a month	2
Less than one headache a month	1

Degree of Disability	Headache Disability Rating (Time Lost Rating × Headache Frequency Rating)
Handicapped	70–121
Severe disability	40–69
Significant disability	30–39
Moderate disability	20–29
Some disability	2–19

Common Headache Triggers

Foods and Food Additives to Avoid	Some Alternatives
Alcohol (particular triggers are Chianti, sherry, Sauternes, Riesling, and beer	
Aspartame, found in artificial sweeteners like NutraSweet, Equal, and in low-calorie processed foods	Sugar, honey
Avocadoes	
Beans: fava, broad, Italian, lima, navy, pinto, garbanzo, lentil, string, and snow peas	Green beans
Breads, such as sourdough, cheese breads, and crackers; hot bread made with yeast	Let hot bread cool before eating

Common Headache Triggers

Foods and Food Additives to Avoid	Some Alternatives
Caffeine	Caffeine in moderate amounts may not act as a trigger
Cheeses (aged): cheddar, Colby, Camembert, Roquefort, Brie, Gruyère, mozzarella, Parmesan, Romano, blue, provolone, Gouda, and Stilton	Cream cheese, American cheese, pot cheese, cottage cheese, Velveeta, and farmer cheeses
Chicken liver, pâté	
Chili peppers	
Chocolate, chocolate milk, cocoa	Jell-O, sherberts, puddings made with skim milk, hard candies, pastries made without chocolate, and pies made with non-trigger fruits (see below)
Coconuts and coconut oil	

Corn	
Dairy products: whole milk, sour cream, homemade yogurt, acidophilus milk, buttermilk, and aged cheeses (*see above*)	Skim milk, 1% or 2% milk, and skim milk–based yogurts in 1/2 cup daily servings
Eggplant	
Fish that has been dried or cured, such as herring, caplin, and cod; also caviar	Tuna fish packed in water and fresh fish
Fried foods	
Fruits (citrus) such as oranges, limes, lemons, tangerines, grapefruit, and pineapples; dried fruits (raisins, figs, and mince-meat blends); bananas, red plums, mangos, papayas, passionfruit, strawberries, and kiwis	Peaches, apples, pears, apricots, prunes, cherries, and fruit cocktail
Licorice	

Common Headache Triggers

Foods and Food Additives to Avoid	Some Alternatives
Meats (cured or processed): lunch meats such as bologna, salami, and pepperoni; hot dogs, bacon, summer sausage; and organ meats, such as kidneys	Fresh and frozen meats
Monosodium glutamate (MSG); hydrolyzed plant protein (HPP) also known as hydrolyzed vegetable protein (HVP); seasoned salt; and meat tenderizer found in prepared foods, commercial gravies and sauces, and frozen dinners	
Nitrites (often used in processed meats and other preserved foods)	
Nuts and seeds (all varieties)	
Olive oil	Butter, margarine, and other cooking oils

Olives	
Onions	
Peanut butter	
Pickles	
Pizza	Pizza may not act as a trigger if you let it cool completely, and then reheat it
Salad dressings	Look for those made without MSG and other triggers
Salt and other products high in sodium	Pepper, other herbs, and white wine vinegar
Seeds, including sunflower, sesame, and pumpkin	
Soups: any canned, bean, cheese; bouillon cubes and packets; and soup mixes flavored with MSG	Check labels for soups that are low in sodium, preservative-free, and don't use MSG

Common Headache Triggers

Foods and Food Additives to Avoid	Some Alternatives
Soy sauce and textured soy protein	
Spinach	
Sulfites, a preservative	
Tomatoes	A 1/2-cup serving or less may not act as a trigger

Environmental Triggers to Avoid

- Altitude changes
- Bright sunlight, irregular light patterns such as sunlight through venetian blinds or light from disco balls, computer monitors, and movie screens
- Loud or constant noise
- Strong odors or fumes or perfume and perfumed products such as scented soaps and potpourri
- Air pollution
- Excessive heat, changes in barometric pressure, strong winds, high humidity, or thunderstorms

Activities That May Act As Triggers

- Exertion: heavy lifting, exercise, coughing, or bowel movements
- Skipping meals
- Traveling in boats, cars, or other vehicles; taking amusement park rides
- Sex
- Sleep: too much sleep (*hypersomnia*), too little sleep (*insomnia*), or sleep disturbances (*sleep apnea, sleep walking, REM sleep*)
- Smoking or inhaling second-hand smoke
- Travel, especially airplane travel across time zones

Psychological Triggers

- Anxiety
- Depression
- Emotional upset (such as that caused by an illness in the family, romantic breakups, work problems, or childrearing)
- Stress
- Tension

Hormonal Changes That May Act as Triggers

- Puberty
- Menstruation
- Birth control pills
- Pregnancy
- Menopause
- Hormone treatments (such as estrogen replacement therapy
- Steroid use

Glossary

abortive drug: a type of medication that relieves headache pain after an attack begins; an abortive drug can be taken at the very first sign of an attack.

acupuncture: a form of physical therapy that orginated in China; it involves placing needles at strategic locations on the body to release natural pain-fighting chemicals.

adrenaline: a hormone released by the body's adrenal glands in response to fear, stress, or some medications; it increases blood flow and may have an impact on migraine.

amine, or **amino acid**: a cluster of three chemicals—carbon, hydrogen, and nitrogen; this compound can be found in the body and in food as well; sometimes they can trigger headache.

analgesic: a type of medication that relieves pain by numbing pain centers.

ancillary disorder: a condition that you have at the same time you're suffering from another separate disorder.

antidepressant: a type of drug used to treat depression; some can be used in the management of migraine.

antiemetic: a medicine that relieves feelings of nausea and stops vomiting.

arteritis (giant cell arteritis): a condition found most often in older patients; it occurs when arteries in the brain become inflamed; if not treated, it can lead to vision loss.

aspartame: a food additive used in artificial sweeteners and in the ingredients of some prepared foods.

aura: visual and perception experiences—such as seeing black spots or flashing lights, having speech or balance problems, feeling numbness in your hands and feet, smelling and hearing things that aren't really there—that appear in the period just before headache pain begins, usually no more than one hour before the headache.

auto-injector: a device that looks like a pen but conceals a needle for injecting medication; the needle descends to pierce the skin when pressure is placed on the injector.

basilar artery migraine: a headache that involves branches of the basilar artery in the brain.

benign: a term used to describe a condition that is not dangerous to your physical health.

beta-blockers: a type of drug originally used in the treatment of high blood pressure, now used for migraine; beta-blockers block the beta receptors that send messages to your brain regulating blood flow.

biofeedback (autogenic training): a technique that patients use to control their bodies' responses by force of concentration and of will, migraineurs learn to raise and lower body temperature levels through training that involves reacting to signals from machines that tell you how well you're doing.

blood pressure: the force of blood pressing against the walls of the arteries and blood vessels as it flows with each pulse.

blood vessels: any vessels (structures) that act as conduits for blood—usually arteries or veins.

brain stem: the part of the brain extending down into the neck; this area contains many serotonin transmitters.

brain tumor: an abnormal growth of cells in the brain; these cells don't serve any known function and interfere with other cell activity.

caffeine: an addictive substance found in coffee, teas, some sodas, and chocolate; it may enhance the effects of migraine medication or act as a trigger.

calcium channel blocker: a type of drug originally used in the treatment of high blood pressure and heart-related conditions; calcium channel blockers block the path of calcium in your body and are now used to manage migraine.

CAT (computerized axial tomography), or **CT scan**: using x-rays to gather images from all different directions, it creates a layered picture of what's happening inside the body; the scans can help spot bleeding in the brain.

cerebellum: part of the brain, located at the base of the skull, right above the back of the neck; it controls coordination, balance—all motor activity.

cerebrum: the familiar crinkled, folded lump of gray cells forming the upper portion of the brain; divided into four lobes and two hemispheres (right and left), it controls memory, emotions, sensory input, and thought.

chronic daily headache: a headache that occurs every day; these are not usually migraine attacks but a combination of tension-type and rebound headaches.

classic migraine: a term used to classify migraine with aura.

classification: a diagnostic method that labels the migraine according to a chart established by the International Headache Society.

cluster headache: a particular kind of headache found most often in male patients; it shows up in regular cycles of several brief headaches a day for a period up to six weeks, this cycle can repeat once or twice a year.

common migraine: this is a term sometimes used to describe migraine without aura; patients usually have no warning of an attack.

compound: a drug or chemical that has more than one basic ingredient.

constrict: to squeeze or shut an opening; many migraine drugs constrict blood vessels so that blood flows with less force.

corticosteroid: an antiinflammatory hormone often used to treat allergies; it also helps in the processing of foods.

diagnosis: a doctor's identification of the disorder, based on a knowledge of its symptoms and effects.

dilate: to widen an opening; it is believed that some of headache's pain is caused by the rush of blood through overly dilated blood vessels in the brain.

disorder: a condition suffered by a patient—an illness, sickness, or disease.

diuretic (water pill): a medication taken to control bloating, such as occurs during a woman's period; diuretics can also be used to treat water retention caused by some migraine treatments.

dopamine: a chemical that helps the nervous system perform its functions, especially in the brain.

Doppler test (transcranial Doppler): a procedure that takes a picture of the inside of the body using ultrasound.

EEG (electroencephalogram): a visual graph of the activity inside the brain; it's generated by sensors attached to the scalp which transmit a picture of what's going on inside.

elimination diet: the controlled intake of food over a period of time, to discover which foods act as trigger; the daily menu is limited to nontrigger foods, then potential triggers are reintroduced one at a time.

endorphins: a chemical produced inside the brain; endorphins create feelings of happiness and are thought to be natural pain-killers.

enzyme: a substance that helps digestion by breaking down proteins, carbohydrates, and fats; enzymes regulate the metabolism in other ways, by creating chemical reactions in the body.

estrogen: a female hormone that aids in a woman's sexual development.

exertional headache: a type of headache that strikes when patients put more-than-normal stress on their bodies, such as when lifting, exercising, or even having sex (known then as orgasmic headache); it's most often experienced by men.

feverfew: an herb, one of the chrysanthemum family, thought to be effective as a preventive for migraine.

first-line defense: the first methods to try in the treatment of migraine, these would include only those drugs approved by the FDA specifically for fighting migraine, and over-the-counter medications.

fortification spectra (teichopsia): a form of visual aura experienced by many headache sufferers, this takes the appearance of a zigzag outline around a darkened center; it looks something like the walls of a fort.

headache: head pain that is a symptom of migraine or some other condition.

headache clinic: a treatment center that may include just one or many doctors, treating the various aspects of migraine—for instance, a clinic may have a neurologist, psychologist, physiotherapist, and nutritionist working together.

headache specialist: a neurologist or other type of doctor dedicated to the treatment of migraine and headache disorders.

hemiplegic migraine (familial hemiplegic migraine): a rare type of migraine found only in sufferers who have a family history of migraine.

histamine: a molecule of the chemical $C_5H_9N_3$, it signals the body that it's being attacked; when large amounts of histamines are released, the body has an allergic reaction; found in aged cheeses and meats, some fish and other foods, histamines are rendered harmless by the liver but may be headache triggers.

history: a medical and lifestyle background taken by a doctor.

hormone: the body's sexual development and the processing of foods are controlled by these substances, which are released by the endocrine glands.

inhibitor: a substance that stops certain chemical or biological actions.

intracranial: literally, "inside the skull."

intranasal: the method of inhaling medications through the nose.

invasive: a procedure involving insertion of an instrument or foreign material into the body; it is sometimes unpleasant or even painful.

ischemia: shutdown of the blood supply to a specific area, sometimes even the heart; it can be caused by misuse of drugs that act as blood vessel constrictors.

IV (intravenous): a method of taking a steady, measured dose of medication, fed directly into the veins, usually through a tube attached to a needle.

macropsia: a type of visual aura that makes people appear stretched out and distorted to a migraineur, or a sufferer may feel oversized themselves; most often experienced by children.

MAO (monoamine oxidase inhibitor): a type of drug originally used to treat depression, now used in some migraine cases, but dangerous when mixed with tyramine in foods.

menstrual migraine: a type of migraine that occurs only in the few days before, during, and after a woman's period, and not at any other time of the month.

micropsia: a visual aura symptom that makes people look small or distorted, or migraineurs may feel as though they themselves have shrunk.

migraine variant (migraine equivalent): a rare type of migraine that does not have head pain as a symptom; instead the pain is centered in the urinary tract or stomach, with nausea and vomiting a symptom.

migraineur: someone who suffers from migraine.

MRI (magnetic resonance imaging): a procedure in which a patient is bombarded with harmless radio waves while enclosed in a magnetic field, usually a large cylinder; the frequencies absorbed by the body allows a computer to create a picture of what's happening inside.

MSG (monosodium glutamate): an additive used in many kinds of foods to enhance flavor, found in a wide variety of canned goods, frozen dinners, and other prepared foods, not just on Chinese menus.

narcotic: a potent drug, usually a prescribed or controlled substance, that relieves pain, dulls the senses, or induces sleep.

negative scotoma: a black spot or area in your field of vision; this is a very common example of aura.

neurologist: a doctor who specializes in the treatment of the nervous system, including the spinal cord and brain.

neurotransmitter: a substance that relays signals back and forth between your brain and the rest of your body; these signals can include messages like ''increase blood flow now!''

nitrite: an additive used to preserve foods, particularly luncheon meats, and a migraine trigger.

NSAID (nonsteroidal antiinflammatory): a drug that acts on inflamed areas of the body; inflammation is the redness, pain, and swelling that occurs when the body sends blood rushing to a spot that has been ''injured'' in some way.

oral: literally, ''in the mouth''; drugs that are swallowed.

OTC (over-the-counter) medication: medicines you can purchase without a prescription.

peptide: a molecule created by the process of digesting proteins, and a possible headache trigger; peptides are found in strawberries, tomatoes, chocolate, and egg whites.

perception disturbance: a symptom experienced by migraineurs all through an attack; any of the senses may be affected.

PET (positive emission tomography) scan: a procedure for looking inside the body that uses an injection of a substance that connects with electrons; this subatomic partnership creates harmless radioactive waves, and machines detect any "hot spots" they show off.

pharmacologic: a drug or medicine; a *nonpharmacologic* treatment would be a therapy that is drug-free.

phonophobia (noise sensitivity): a common symptom of migraine that causes a sufferer to find the slightest sound too painful and loud to bear.

photophobia (light sensitivity): a symptom of migraine; patients find it painful to look at anything from bright sunshine to even very dim light.

photopsia: a form of visual aura that looks like shooting stars of light.

post-traumatic headache: pain that follows a blow or other accident to the head.

present: a term used by doctors to mean the symptoms described or demonstrated by a patient.

preventive drugs: a type of medication taken every day to stop headaches from starting.

prodrome: the period of time right before a headache, defined by warning signs such as aura, dizziness, or nausea that may show up minutes or hours before pain strikes.

progesterone: a female hormone that prepares the body for pregnancy.

progressive relaxation: a method of releasing tight muscles, one group at a time.

prophylactic: an agent used to prevent disease.

prophylaxis: the prevention of disease.

prostaglandin: chemicals similar to hormones, released by the body.

rebound headache: a daily headache that's caused by the overuse of medicines.

referred pain: a pain signal that seems to come from one area but is actually related to another place in your body; for example, the numb arm felt during a heart attack.

refractory headache: a headache that's especially painful or lasts longer than usual, or headache attacks that strike every day.

rescue medication: a drug taken when an attack is in progress; it may not work if used as a preventive.

reward system: a cycle created when your body becomes addicted to a drug and the feeling, or reward, that medication can deliver.

scotoma: bright-colored lines that show up during aura or even during an attack; *scintillating scotoma* are bright flashing lights or wavy lines.

second-line defense: the second set of options to try when treating migraine, including drugs not yet approved by the FDA for migraine, although they might be approved for the treatment of other disorders, such as high blood pressure.

serotonin (5-hydroxytryptamine, 5-HT): a neurotransmitter that carries messages from one cell to the next; it's thought to have a role in sleep cycles of alertness and drowsiness and so is considered a player in headache pain.

sinusitis: an infection or blockage in the sinus area behind the nose, forehead, and eyes.

spinal tap (lumbar puncture): a medical procedure performed in hospitals; a needle is used to remove spinal fluid so that the pressure can be measured and other information determined from the cell count.

steroid: a type of antiinflammatory drug sometimes used in the treatment of migraine; steroids can have unpleasant and sometimes dangerous side effects

subcutaneous: literally, "under the skin"; this term refers to drugs that are injected beneath the surface of your skin.

sublingual: literally, "under the tongue"; in migraine it's used to describe medicines that are dissolved under the tongue.

symptom: a signal that something is wrong inside the body; headache pain, visual disturbances, numbness, slurred speech, and cold fingers can all be symptoms.

tension-type headache: the most common type of headache, not considered migraine because it doesn't have aura, light sensitivity, or nausea symptoms; it's thought to be caused by tightened muscles in the head, neck, and shoulders.

third-line defense: this is a set of treatment options that should only be tried after first- and second-line defense methods have failed; they include narcotics and drugs with potentially disturbing or dangerous side effects.

TMJ (temporomandibular joint) syndrome: a condition centered on the area around the jaw and mouth joints.

tricyclic antidepressant: a type of drug used to treat depression but also taken for migraine; tricyclic antidepressants stop the action of serotonin.

trigeminal nerve: a bundle of nerves that relay sensory messages, like pain, from areas of the face.

trigger: something that sets off an attack, including food, a behavior pattern, a situation, or something that you see, smell, or hear.

trigger point: an area of the body feeling pain; *trigger point injection therapy* involves piercing these areas with needles to release the body's natural pain-fighting chemicals.

tyramine: a headache-triggering chemical classified as an amine, found in some foods, especially those that are aged, like cheese and wine.

unilateral: literally "one-sided"; in migraine this refers to headache pain on only one side of the head, although the location can shift from one attack to the next, or even during an attack.

vascular: relating in some way to the flow of blood through the blood vessels.

vasoactive: having an effect on the blood vessels, either squeezing them shut or opening them wide.

Bibliography

Chapter 1

Ad Hoc Committee on Classification of Headache. "Classification of Headache." *The Journal of the American Medical Association*, 1962, *179*, 717–718.

Headache Classification Committee of the International Headache Society. "Classification and Diagnostic Criteria for Headache Disorders, Cranial Neuralgias and Facial Pain." *Cephalalgia*, 1988, *8* (Suppl. 7), 1–96.

Hopkins, S. and Ziegler, D. K. "Headache—The size of the problem." In Hopkins, A. (Ed.), *Headache: Problems in Diagnosis and Management*. London: W. B. Saunders Company, 1988.

Linet, M. S., Stewart, W. F., and Celentano, D. D., *et al.* "An epidemiological study of headache among adolescents and young adults." *Journal of the American Medical Association*, 1989, *26*, 2211–2216.

Stewart, W. F., Lipton, R. B., and Celentano, D. D., *et al.* "The epidemiology of severe migraine headaches from a national survey: Implications of projections to the United States population." *Cephalalgia*, 1991, *11* (Suppl. 11), 87–88.

Stewart, W. R., Lipton, R. B., Celentano, D. D., and Reed, M. L. "Prevalence of migraine headache in the United States." *Journal of the American Medical Association*, 1992, *267* (No. 1), 64–69.

Ulrich, O. *Headache and Migraine Answers*. Online: http://ourworld.compuserve.com/homepages/Ulrich_Oswald/.

Ziegler, D. K. "The contribution of epidemiology to the understanding of headache and migraine." In Hopkins, A. (Ed.), *Headache: Problems in Diagnosis and Management*. London: W. B. Saunders Company, 1988.

Chapter 2

Diamond, S. and Dalessio, D. J. "Classification and mechanism of headache." In Diamond, S. & Dalessio, D.J. (Eds.), *The Practicing Physician's Approach to Headache* (5th ed.). Baltimore: Williams and Wilkins, 1992.

Graham, J. G. "Cluster headache and pain in the face." In Hopkins, A. (Ed.), *Problems in Diagnosis and Management*. Philadelphia: W. B. Saunders Company, 1988.

Hay, K. "The assessment of disability caused by migraine." *The Practitioner*, 1989, *233*, 573–574.

Kudrow, L. "Treatment of cluster headache." *Headache Quarterly*, 1993, *4* (Suppl. 2), 42–47.

Kunkel, R. S. "Diagnosis and treatment of muscle contraction (tension-type) headaches." In Diamond, S. (Ed.), *Medical Clinics of North America* (Vol. 75[3]). Philadelphia: W. B. Saunders Company, 1991.

Lachman, B. *The Journal of Hildegard of Bingen*. New York: Bell Tower, 1993.

Lerman, K. *The Life and Works of Hildegard von Bingen (1098–1179)*. Online: http://www.netspot.unisa.edu.au/pt/migraine.html.

Mathew, N. T. "Advances in cluster headache." In Mathew, N. T. (Ed.), *Neurologic Clinics* (Vol. 8[4]). Philadelphia: W. B. Saunders Company, 1990.

Panayiotopoulos, C. P. "Elementary visual hallucinations in migraine and epilepsy." *Journal of Neurology, Neurosurgery and Psychiatry,* 1994, *57,* 1371–1374.

Sacks, O. *Migraine, Revised and Expanded.* London: Faber and Faber, 1991.

Von Bingen, H. *Mystical Visions.* Introduction by Matthew Fox. Santa Fe: Bear & Company Publishing, 1986.

Chapter 3

Block, P. McL. "Medical progress: Brain tumors." *New England Journal of Medicine,* 1991, *324*(21-22), 1471–1476, 1555–1564.

Dalessio, D. J. "Pain-sensitive structures within the cranium." In Dalessio, D. J. (Ed.), *Wolff's Headache and Other Head Pain* (4th ed.). New York: Oxford University Press, 1980.

Diamond, S. and Dalessio, D. J. "Classification and mechanism of headache." In Diamond, S. and Dalessio, D. J. (Eds.), *The Practicing Physician's Approach to Headache* (5th ed.). Baltimore: Williams and Wilkins, 1992.

Edmeads, J. "Headaches and head pains associated with disease of the cervical spine." *Medical Clinics of North America,* 1978, *62,* 533–544.

Elkind, A. H., Friedman, A. P., and Grossman, J. "Cutaneous blood flow in vascular headaches of the migraine type." *Neurology,* 1964, *14* (No. 1), 24–29.

Goodman, B. W. "Temporal Arteritis." *American Journal of Medicine,* 1979, *67,* 839–852.

Graham, J. R. and Wolff, H. G. "Mechanisms of migraine and action of ergotamine tartrate." *Archives of Neurology and Psychology*, 1938, *39*, 737–763.

Heyck, H. (Ed.). *Headache and Facial Pain. Differential Diagnosis-Pathogenesis-Treatment.* Chicago: Year Book Medical Publishers, Inc., 1981.

Hobson, J. A. *Sleep.* New York: Scientific American Library, 1989.

Humphrey, P. P. A. "5-Hydroxytrytamine and the pathophysiology of migraine." *Journal of Neurology*, 1991, *238*, S38–S34.

Lance, J. W. (Ed.). *Mechanism and Management of Headache* (5th ed.). Oxford: Butterworth-Heinemann, 1993.

Lance, J. W., Anthony, M., and Hinterberger, H. "The control of cranial arteries by humoral mechanisms and its relation to the migraine syndrome." *Headache*, 1967, *7*, 93–102.

Moskowitz, M. A. "Neurobiology of vascular head pain." *Annals of Neurology*, 1984, *16*, 157–168.

Raskin, N. H., Hosobuchi, Y., and Lamb, J. "Headache may arise from perturbation of the brain." *Headache*, 1987, *27*, 416–420.

Ray, B. S., and Wolff, H. G. "Experimental studies on headache: pain-sensitive structures of the head and their significance in headache." *Archives of Surgery*, 1940, *41*, 813–856.

Rosenblum, B. N., and Friedman, W. H. "Paranasal sinus etiologies of headache and facial pain." In Jacobson, A.L. and Donlon, W.C. (Eds.), *Headache and Facial Pain. Diagnosis and Management.* New York: Raven Press, 1990.

Russell, R. W. R. and Graham, E. M. "Giant Cell Arteritis." In Hopkins, A. (Ed.), *Headache: Problems in Diagnosis and Management.* Philadelphia: W. B. Saunders Company, 1988.

Tomsak, R. L. "Ophthalmologic aspects of headache." In Diamond, S. (Ed.), *Medical Clinics of North America* (Vol. 75[3]). Philadelphia: W. B. Saunders Company, 1991.

Welch, K. M. A., D'Amdrea, G., Tepley, N., Barkley, G., and Ramadan, N. M. "The concept of migraine as a state of central neuronal hyperexcitability." In Mathew, N. T. (Ed.), *Neurologic Clinics* (Vol. 8[4]). Philadelphia: W. B. Saunders Company, 1990.

Chapter 4

Anthony, M. and Lance, J. W. "Monoamine oxidase inhibition in the treatment of migraine." *Archives of Neurology*, 1969, *21*, 263–268.

Diamond, S. "Migraine Headaches." In Diamond, S. (Ed.), *Medical Clinics of North America* (Vol. 75[3]). Philadelphia: W. B. Saunders, 1991.

Elkind, A. H. "Drug abuse in headache patients." *Clinical Journal of Pain*, 1989, *5*, 111–120.

Elkind, A. H. "Provoking influences in migraine: The controversies." In Saper, J. R. (Ed.), *Controversies and Clinical Variants of Migraine*. New York: Pergamon Press, 1987.

Gibb, C. M., Davies, P. T. G., Glover, V., Steiner, T. J., Rose, F. C., and Sandler, M. "Chocolate is a migraine-provoking agent." *Cephalalgia*, 1991, *11*, 93–95.

Gilliland, K. and Bullock, W. "Caffeine: A potential drug of abuse." *Advances in Alcohol and Substance Abuse*, 1983, *3*, 53–73.

Hobson, J. A. *Sleep*. New York: Scientific American Library, 1989.

Jacobson, M. F. and Maxwell, B. *What Are We Feeding Our Kids?* New York: Workman Publishing, 1994.

Littlewood, J. T., Gibb, C., Glover, V., Sandler, M., Davies, P. T. G., and Rose, F. C. "Red wine as a cause of migraine." *Lancet*, 1988, *8585*, 558–559.

Marlin, J. T. and Bertelli, D. *The Catalogue of Healthy Food: On Farms, In Stores and Restaurants*. New York: Bantam Books, 1990.

Potera, C. "Exercise moderates migraine." *American Health*, 1994, *13*, 96.

Sahota, P. K. and Dexter, J. D. "Sleep and headache syndromes: A clinical review." *Headache*, 1990, *30*, 1990: 80–84.

Vaugh, T. R. "The role of food in the pathogenesis of migraine." *Clinical Review of Allergy*, 1994, *12*(2), 167–180.

Weiss, B. "Food additive safety evaluation." *Advances in Child Psychology*, 1984, *7*, 221–251.

Chapter 5

Dalton, K. "Migraine and oral contraceptives." *Headache*, 1975, *15*, 247.

Gallagher, R. M. "Menstrual migraine and intermittent ergonovine therapy." *Headache*, 1989, *29*, 366–367.

Kirkcaldy, B. D., Kobylinska, E., and Furnham, A.F. "MMPI profiles of male and female migraine sufferers." *Social Science and Medicine*, 1993, *37*, 879–882.

Silberstein, S. D. "Headaches in women: Treatment of the pregnant and lactating migraineur." *Headache*, 1993, *33*, 533-540.

Solbach, M. P., & Waymer, R. S. "Treatment of menstruation-associated migraine headache with subcutaneous sumatriptan." *Obstetrics and Gynecology*, 1993, *82*(5), 769–772.

Chapter 6

Deskin, G. and Steckler, G. *The Parent's Answer Book*. Minneapolis: Fairview Press, 1996.

Gilbert, C. "Coping with pediatric migraine." *Child and Adolescent Social Work Journal*, 1995, *12*, 275–287.

Kuttner, L. *A Child in Pain: How To Help, What To Do*. Point Roberts: Hartley & Marks Publishers, 1996.

Lascelles, M. A., Cunningham, S. J., McGrath, P., and Sullivan, M. J. L. "Helping adolescents manage migraine headaches." *American Journal of Nursing*, 1989, *89*, 1215–1216.

Lundberg, P. O. "Abdominal migraine—Diagnosis and therapy." *Headache*,1995, *15*, 122–125.

Markel, H. and Oski, F.A. *The Practical Pediatrician*. New York: W. H. Freeman, 1995.

Rothner, A. D. "Headache syndromes in children and adolescents: Diagnosis and management." In Diamond, S. and Dalessio, D. J. (Eds.), *The Practicing Physician's Approach to Headache* (5th ed.). Baltimore: Williams and Wilkins, 1992.

Chapter 7

Cady, R. K. "The role of family physicians in migraine management." *Headache Quarterly*, 1993, *4*(Suppl. 2), 21–28.

Diamond, M. L. "Emergency department treatment of the headache patient." *Headache Quarterly*, 1992, *3*(Suppl. 1), 28–33.

Diamond, S. and Dalessio, D. J. (Eds.). *The Practicing Physician's Approach to Headache* (5th ed.). Baltimore: Williams and Wilkins, 1992.

Prager, J. M. and Mikulis, D. J. "The radiology of headache.'' In Diamond, S. (Ed.), *Medical Clinics of North America*. Philadelphia: W. B. Saunders Company, 1991.

van Dijk, J. G. "No confirmation of visual-evoked potential diagnostic test for migraine." *Lancet*, 1991, *337*, 517–518.

Chapter 8

Anthony, M., and Lance, J. W. "Monoamine oxidase inhibition in the treatment of migraine." *Archives of Neurology*, 1969, *21*, 263–268.

Behan, P. O. and Connelly, K. "Prophylaxis of migraine: A comparison between naproxen sodium and pizotifen." *Headache*, 1986, *26*, 237.

Blau, J. N. "Neurobiology and migraine." In Blau, J.N. (Ed.), *Migraine—Clinical and Research Aspects*. Baltimore: John Hopkins University Press, 1987.

Bristol-Myers Squibb. *Stadol NS* (Product Monograph). Princeton, 1992.

Buring, J. E., Peto, R., and Hennekens, C. H. "Low-dose aspirin for migraine prophylaxis." *Journal of the American Medical Association*, 1990, *264*, 1711.

Cady, R. K. "United States Experience with Sumatriptan." *Headache Quarterly*, 1993, *4*(Suppl.), 29–33.

Cady, R. K., Wendt, J. K., Kirchner, J. R., Sargent, J. D., Rothrock, J. F., and Skaggs, H., Jr. "Treatment of acute migraine with subcutaneous sumatriptan." *Journal of the American Medical Association*, 1991, *265*(21), 2831–2835.

Carolei, A., Marini, C., De Mattels, G., and the Italian National Research Council Study Group on Stroke in the Young. "History of migraine and risk of cerebral ischemia in young adults." *Lancet*, 1996, *347*, 1503–1506.

The Cluster Headache Study Group. "Treatment of acute

cluster headache with Sumatriptan.'' *New England Journal of Medicine*, 1991, *325*(5), 322–326.

Couch, J. R., Ziegler, D. K., and Hassanein, R. ''Amitriptyline in the prophylaxis of migraine: Effectiveness and relationship of antimigraine and antidepressant drugs.'' *Neurology*, 1976, *26*, 121–127.

Dalessio, D. J. ''Prophylactic treatment of headache.'' *Headache Quarterly*, 1993, *4*(Suppl. 2), 12–20.

Diamond, S., Freitag, F. G., Diamond, M. L., and Urban, G. ''Transnasal butorphanol in the treatment of migraine pain.'' *Headache Quarterly*, 1992, *3*(2), 160–166.

Ekbom, K. ''Lithium for cluster headache: Review of the literature and preliminary results of long-term treatments.'' *Headache*, 1981, *21*, 132–139.

Elkind, A. H. ''Additional pharmaceutical agents used in migraine prophylaxis.'' In Diamond, S. (Ed.), *Migraine Headache Prevention and Management*. New York: Marcel Dekker, 1990.

Elkind, A. H. ''Drug abuse and headache.'' In *Medical Clinics of North America* (Vol. 75). Philadelphia: W. B. Saunders Company, 1991.

Elkind, A. H. ''Interval therapy of migraine: The art and science.'' *Headache Quarterly*, 1990, *1*, 280–289.

Elkind, A. H. ''Matching dosage forms to the needs of your headache patient.'' *Headache Quarterly*, 1992, *3*(Suppl. 1), 16–21.

Elkind, A. H. ''The acute treatment of migraine.'' *Headache Quarterly*, 1993, *4*(Suppl.), 4–11.

Elkind, A. H. ''The use of narcotics in the treatment of headache.'' *Headache Quarterly*, 1993, *4*(2), 143–144.

Elkind, A. H., Chu, G., and Diamond, S. "Evaluation of the safety and efficacy of transnasal butorphanol in the treatment of acute migraine in outpatients." *Abstract: 9th Migraine Trust International Symposium.* London, 1992.

Elkind, A. H. and Indelicato, J. "A retrospective study with divalproex sodium for refractory headache prophylaxis." *Headache Quarterly*, 1994, *5*, 149–152.

Friberg, L., Olesen, J., Iverson, H. K., and Sperling, B. "Migraine pain associated with middle cerebral artery dilation: Reversal by sumatriptan." *Lancet*, 1991, *338*, 13–17.

Friedman, A. P. and Elkind, A. H. "Appraisal of methysergide in treatment of vascular headaches of migraine type." *Journal of the American Medical Association*, 1963, *184*, 125–128.

Gallagher, R. M. "Proper use of analgesics in the treatment of headache." *Headache Quarterly*, 1992, *3*(Suppl. 1), 22–27.

Goadsby, P. J., Zagami, A. S., Donnan, G. A., Symington, G., Anthony, M., Bladin, P. F., and Lance, J. W. "Oral sumatriptan in acute migraine." *Lancet*, 1991, *338*(8770), 782–783.

Graham, J. "Cardiac and pulmonary fibrosis during methysergide therapy for migraine." *American Journal of Medical Science*, 1967, *257*, 1–12.

Havanka-Kannianen, H. "Treatment of acute migraine attack: Ibuprofen and placebo compared." *Headache*, 1989, *29*, 507.

Heathfield, K. W. G., Stone, P., and Crowder, D. "Pizotifen in the treatment of migraine." *The Practitioner*, 1977, *218*, 428–430.

Hosman-Benjaminse, S. L. and Bolhuis, P. A. "Migraine and

platelet aggregation in patients treated with low-dose acety-salicyclic acid.'' *Headache*, 1986, *26*, 282–284.

Klapper, J. A. ''Recent advances in the treatment of cluster headache.'' *Headache Quarterly*, 1992, *3*(Suppl. 1), 10–15.

Kudrow, L.''Lithium prophylaxis for chronic cluster headache.'' *Headache*, 1977, *17*, 15–18.

Lehne, R. A., in consultation with Moore, L. A., Crosby, L. J., and Hamilton, D. B. *Pharmacology for Nursing Care* (2nd ed.). Philadelphia: W. B. Saunders Company, 1994.

Markley, H. G. ''Verapamil and migraine prophylaxis: Mechanisms and efficacy.'' *American Journal of Medicine*, 1991, *90*(Suppl. 5A), 48–53.

Mathew, N. ''Clinical subtypes of cluster headache and response to lithium therapy.'' *Headache*, 1978, *18*, 26–80.

Mathew, N. T. and Sanin, L. C. ''Advances in migraine drug therapy.'' *Drug Therapy*, 1993 March, 37–48.

Meyer, J. S. ''Calcium blockers in the prophylactic treatment of vascular headache.'' *Annals of Internal Medicine*, 1985, *102*, 395–397.

Mondell, B. E. ''Office management of acute headache.'' *Headache Quarterly*, 1992, *3*(Suppl. 1), 4–9.

Nestvoid, K., Kloster, R., and Partinen, M., *et al.* ''Treatment of acute migraine attack: Naproxen and placebo compared.'' *Cephalalgia*, 1985, *5*, 115.

O'Neill, B. P. and Mann, J. D. ''Aspirin prophylaxis in migraine.'' *Lancet*, 1978, *2*, 1179-1181.

Peatfield, R. C. ''Migraine—Unproven Therapeutic Measures.'' In Diamond, S. (Ed.), *Migraine Headache Prevention and Management*. New York: Marcel Dekker, 1990.

Peters, B., Fraim, C. J., and Masel, B. E. ''Comparison of

650 mg aspirin and 1000 mg acetaminophen with each other and with placebo in moderately severe headache." *American Journal of Medicine*, June 14, 1983, 36–42.

Rall, T. W., "Hypnotics and sedatives: Ethanol." In Gilman, A. G., Rall, T. W., Nies, A. S., and Taylor, P. (Eds.), *Goodman & Gilman's The Pharmacological Basis of Therapeutics* (8th ed.). Elmsford, N.Y.: Pergamon Press, 1990.

Raskin, N. H. *Headache* (2nd ed.). New York: Churchill-Livingstone, 1988.

Raskin, N. H. "Repetitive intravenous dihydroergotamine as therapy for intractable migraine." *Neurology*, 1986, *36*, 1995.

Raskin, N. H. "Modern pharmacotherapy of migraine." In Mathew, N.T. (Ed.), *Neurologic Clinics* (Vol. 8[4]). Philadelphia: W. B. Saunders Company, 1990.

Rose, F. C. "Sumatriptan: An overview." *Headache Quarterly*, 1993, *4* (Suppl. 2), 37–41.

Saper, J. and Silberstein, S. "Safety and efficacy of divalproex sodium in the prophylaxis of migraine headache: A multi-center, double-blind, placebo-controlled trial." *Neurology*, 1993, *43*, A401.

Sargent, J. D., Baumel, B., and Peters, K., *et al*. "Aborting a migraine attack: Naproxen sodium vs. ergotamine plus caffeine." *Headache*, 1988, *28*, 263.

Siulc, E. "Elsa's Page: University of Pittsburgh." Migraine headaches. Online: *elsst21+@pitt.eu*.

Skaer, T. L. "Clinical presentation and treatment of migraine." *Clinical Therapeutics*, 1996, *18*(2), 229–241.

Solomon, G. D., Steel, J. G., and Spaccavento, L. J. "Verapamil prophylaxis of migraine: A double-blind, placebo-controlled study." *Journal of the American Medical Association*, 1983, *250*, 2500–2502.

Speed, W. G. "Treatment of muscle contraction (tension) headache." In *Gallagher, R. M. (Ed.), Drug Therapy for Headache*. New York: Marcel Dekker, 1990.

The Subcutaneous Sumatriptan International Study Group. "Treatment of migraine attacks with sumatriptan." *New England Journal of Medicine*, 1991, *325*(5), 316–321.

Turkewitz, L. J., Casaly, J. S., Dawson, G. A., and Wirth, O. "Phenelzine therapy for headache patients with concomitant depression and anxiety." *Headache*, 1992, *32*, 203–207.

Ziegler, D. K. and Ellis, D. J. "Naproxen sodium in prophylaxis of migraine." *Archives of Neurology*, 1985, *42*, 582.

Chapter 9

Blanchard, E. B., Applebaum, K. A., and Guarnieri, P., *et al.* "Five-year prospective follow-up on the treatment of chronic headache with biofeedback and/or relaxation." *Headache*, 1987, *27*, 580–583.

Blumenthal, D. "Massage goes mainstream." *American Health*, 1991, *10*, 68–71.

Brown, D. J. "Manage migraines naturally." *Let's Live*, 1995, *63*, 50–53.

Diamond, S. "Exercise and headaches." Physician and Sports Medicine, 1994, *19*, 78–94.

Dolan, E. F. *Folk Medicine Cures & Curiosities*. New York: Ivy Books, 1993.

Duckro, P. N. "Biofeedback in the management of headache, Part 1." *Headache Quarterly*, 1992, *1*(4), 290–298.

Foster, Steven. "Feverfew." *Better Nutrition for Today's Living*, 1995, *57*, 74–77.

Hudzinski, L. G. and Levenson, H. "Biofeedback behavioral treatment of headache with locus of control pain analysis: A 20-month retrospective study." *Headache*, 1985, *25*, 380–386.

Kasper, S. "Attitude adjustment: Doctors are learning that meditation and other alternatives can help heal." *The Kansas City Star*, December 17, 1995.

Mauskop, A. "Magnesium and headaches." *NHF Head Lines*, Spring 1996, No. 96.

"Migraine headache may respond to feverfew." *Better Nutrition for Today's Living*, 1995, *57*, 26.

Munson, M. "Nature's Head Healer?" *Prevention*, 1995, *47*, 48–50.

Ottoson, D. and Laudenberg, T. (Eds.). *Pain Treatment. A Practical Manual by Transcutaneous Electrical Nerve Stimulation*. Berlin: Springer-Verlag, 1988.

Peterson, N. *Herbs and Health*. Devon, England: Webb & Bower, 1989.

Reese, K. M. "Ancient skulls may hold clues to form of surgery." *Chemical and Engineering News*, 1990, *68*, 94.

Sargent, J. D., Green, E. E., and Walters, E. D. "The use of autogenic feedback training in a pilot study of migraine and tension headaches." *Headache*, 1972, *12*, 120.

St. John Kelly, E. "Healing touches: New respect for alternative medicine." *The Buffalo News*, February 6, 1996.

Chapter 10

Jenkinson, C. "Health status and mood state in a migraine sample." *International Journal of Social Psychiatry*, Spring 1990, *36*, 42–48.

Kohler, T. and Haimerl, C. "Daily stress as a trigger of migraine attacks." *Journal of Consulting and Clinical Psychology*, 1990, *58*, 870–872.

Sachs, J. S. "A fix for migraine." *Health*, Jan.-Feb. 1996, 86–88.

Solberg, R. "*Ronda's Migraine Page*." Online: http://www.ntek.com/ronda.

Beyond This Book:
Resources for Headache Sufferers

There are many resources you can turn to for help as you struggle with migraine—you just need to know where to look. This section will direct you to organizations that can provide information and treatment referrals, as well as hook you up with local support groups. There are some tips for using the Internet to find help and connect with distant sufferers. Finally, I've listed additional books on the subject of migraine and its treatment, which you can use to expand your headache library.

ORGANIZATIONS THAT CAN HELP
There are a number of migraine organizations and foundations out there, most of which are reputable, caring groups that act as patient advocates. The best ones have strong regional support systems to help you find the best care possible. Others have no credentials and, despite good intentions, may be generating information that is out of date or inaccurate. So try the ones listed here and ask for referrals to branches or affiliated groups closer to home.

National Headache Foundation (NHF)

428 W. St. James Place, 2nd Floor
Chicago, IL 60614-2750
(312) 388-6399
Headache Hotline: 1-800-843-2256

FAX (312) 525-7357
Monday-Friday, 9:00 a.m. to 5:00 p.m. CT
Website address: *http://www.headaches.org/*

The National Headache Foundation is the oldest and largest organization serving migraine sufferers. The foundation describes itself this way: A volunteer, nonprofit organization, established by a group of physicians to assist headache sufferers and healthcare professionals, and to increase public awareness about the debilitating nature of headaches. The foundation is dedicated to three major goals.

1. To serve as an information resource to headache sufferers, their families, and the physicians who treat them.
2. To promote research into potential headache causes and treatments.
3. To educate the public to the fact that headaches are serious disorders, and sufferers need understanding and continuity of care.

To meet those goals, NHF provides free information on headache, holds classes for both patients and doctors, and contributes money to headache research. It produces materials for headache sufferers; some of them are listed below. Even people who aren't members of NHF can benefit from its network of support groups.

You may write to the NHF for informational brochures on migraine and for recommendations of specialists. When writing for information, include a brief description of the kind of headache or migraine you suffer from. If you're not sure which type you have, simply list your symptoms. The NHF will tailor the information they send to fit. Be sure to ask for a list of physicians; they'll provide a list of those in your state who are NHF members. The foundation won't suggest just one doctor, but will give *you* the option of choosing by directing you to a number of doctors. Provide a self-addressed envelope, posted with three first-class stamps. Your doctor may also request a copy of the foundation's Therapeutic Guide, a list of all drugs found to be of value in the treatment of headache.

The National Headache Foundation currently has twenty thousand members, 1,500 of whom are physicians or other health-care professionals; the rest of the number is made up of migraineurs and their supporters. Membership to NHF includes four issues of the *NHF Head Lines* newsletter each year, a mailing of brochures from the list below, access to NHF information services, and listings of support groups in your area. As noted, you may also request a list of local NHF physician members. The foundation also sponsors a number of public awareness seminars on migraine each year. These are led by a team of doctors who update the audience on the latest treatment options and answer questions from the floor. Call and ask about this year's schedule.

The National Headache Foundation's support group network is a valuable source of information and strength for headache sufferers; get a list of contact names for your state. If there isn't a support group in your area, and you'd like to start one yourself, call Ellen Blau, NHF's Support Group Coordinator, at 1-800-372-7742.

The NHF's website has general information about the foundation, provides an e-mail membership application, and has a form for ordering from a list of more than thirty fact sheets on a range of headache and migraine subjects. The site also features up-to-date locations of support groups, along with contact names and excerpts from recent meetings.

Here are some of the helpful materials available through the NHF, all of which can be ordered through their websites:

- *The Headache Chart*, which lists twenty-one different types of headaches, their symptoms, precipitating factors, treatment, and prevention.
- *The Headache Handbook*, a brochure filled with general information on causes and types of headaches as well as treatments available.
- *About Headaches*, another brochure, taking a more in-depth look at headaches and treatment.
- *The Relaxation Tape*, an audiocassette detailing relaxation and self-control techniques, broken down into thirty-minute and fifteen-minute exercises.
- *Stretch and Relax Tape*, a second cassette, featuring

exercises that use progressive relaxation, visualization, and imagery techniques.
- *How To Talk To Your Doctor*, a pamphlet that will help guide interactions with medical staff, with tips on your role in the doctor-patient relationship.
- *Headache Q&A*, frequently asked questions and answers about headache and migraine are printed on an easy-access card.
- *No More Headaches*, a videocassette that looks at causes, triggers, procedures, new treatments, and lifestyle solutions.
- *Headache and Diet: Tyramine-Free Recipes*, a spiral-bound recipe book of invaluable aid to sufferers with tyramine triggers.
- *The Hormone Headache*, a book for those with menstrual migraine and other hormone-related headache.

American Association for the Study of Headache (AASH)

This association is made up of hundreds of physicians, health professionals, and research scientists, many of whom contribute to the articles appearing in the organization's newsletter. AASH physicians also answer questions sent to them in the newsletter and provide information to patients through ACHE's electronic support network. The association sponsors a number of educational programs throughout the year and develops materials available to physicians treating migraine. That makes it a valuable resource for your doctor, who can use it to get the most up-to-date information to apply to your care. But for migraineurs, AASH is of interest primarily for its connection to the sister group, ACHE, described below.

American Council for Headache Education (ACHE)
875 Kings Highway, Suite 200
Woodbury, NJ 08096-3172
(609) 845-0322
1-800-255-ACHE (2243)

FAX (609) 384-5811
Website address: *http://www.achenet.org/*

ACHE describes itself as a nonprofit patient/health-professional partnership dedicated to advancing the treatment and management of headache and to raising the public awareness of headache as a valid, biologically based illness.

That means the organization works with both halves of the migraine equation: patients and their doctors. They don't offer specific medical advice but direct you to the people and places that will give you proper care. If you're not happy with your current medical care, contact this organization and request a list of AASH physician members close to you. You can also ask for tips on how to choose the right one to serve your needs.

ACHE's stated goal is to help patients become informed partners in their own care. One way they support this aim is through the organization's newsletter, *Headache*, published four times each year and mailed to members. Issues are a fund of information on migraine; migraineurs who aren't members should check their local libraries for recent issues.

Membership in ACHE costs $15 per year and is considered a tax-deductible donation. In additional to the newsletter, members receive other ACHE materials and information. ACHE organizes support groups nationwide as well as a variety of information and support services online.

ACHE publishes a number of brochures, available through written requests or by using their fax-back system. Call the toll-free number for instructions and a list of the materials.

Many patients use ACHE to find local support groups. ACHE believes that contact with other sufferers is an important element in the treatment of migraine. As they put it, "Besides offering a forum for information exchange, support groups build self-esteem by allowing you to validate your personal experiences with others who accept and understand." Call the toll-free number to get locations, or visit ACHE'S website.

Online, you can find ACHE-sponsored libraries, migraine health forums, message boards, question-and-answer bulletin boards, and "live" events in chat rooms on America Online, CompuServe, and Prodigy. ACHE also has its own website on the Internet which displays enrollment information, schedules for online events, support group listings and contact names, and background materials on the organization.

MIGRAINEURS IN CANADA SHOULD CONTACT

The Migraine Foundation (Canada)
120 Carlton Street, Suite 210
Toronto, Ontario M5A 4K2
(416) 920-4916; 1-800-663-3557
24-hour info line (416) 920-4917
Website addresses: *http://www.tph.ca/wwwpages/charityp/migraine.htm*

MIGRAINEURS OVERSEAS SHOULD CONTACT

The British Migraine Association
178A High Road
Byfleet, Surrey, KT14 7ED
Help line: 011-44-1932-352468

INTERNET GUIDELINES

There is currently some controversy about the value of medical information found on the Internet and through commercial online service providers. You should certainly be cautious about any suggestions and recommendations you find online. Some medical choices, while presented with the best intentions, are simply not sound. Others may be cleverly disguised sales pitches. Take suggestions and stories with a grain of salt even if they come from a reputable source, and discuss new therapies discovered online with your doctor.

Online sites might be of the most value by providing a network of support and encouragement. They connect with migraine-themed ''newsgroups'' and ''chat rooms.'' Newsgroups are areas where people can post and answer questions; some of these exchanges occur in real time. Chat rooms are places where you can enter an ongoing conversation about migraine—or any other subject under the sun. These online sites let sufferers talk with other people who have migraine. Sometimes this comfort from strangers is a much-needed boost to morale. People living in remote areas, where real-life support groups aren't an option, may find it easier to link up with a "virtual" version. Some migraineurs have created home pages, where they post information, share stories, and provide links to other areas of interest to headache sufferers. Here are some online sites to try.

Ronda's Home Page

http://www.ntek.com/ronda
This page is of value not just for the links it provides to other online sites focused on migraine—saving *you* the effort of hunting around—but also for Ronda's upbeat, encouraging attitude to the disorder. You'll find the stories and histories of dozens of other migraineurs, many of which may ring a bell. There are also interviews with headache specialists, answers to questions posted by sufferers, drug lists, artwork relating to migraine, chat room links, and an ongoing reader survey. You'll also find reams of well-meaning advice and suggestions to take back to your own doctor.

FAQs

http://www.social.com/health/faqs.html
For a list of frequently asked questions (FAQs) on the subject of migraine, try the address above or access this site through Ronda's home page. Check the date the FAQ document was updated to make sure it's a recent version of this document, which is changed periodically. Much of the information it provides is covered in this book in broader detail, but it's a good basic introduction to the world of migraine concerns. There may be several FAQ documents listed.

Newsgroups

alt.support.headaches.migraine
Newsgroups are places where people can exchange information by posting questions and answering one another. The information provided here is anecdotal and should therefore be discussed with your doctor.

Search Words

There are places online where the job of hunting for information on specific subjects has been done for you. These are called "search engines." Some of the most well-known are Altavista, Excite, WebCrawler, and Yahoo. Once in a search engine, enter migraine-related search words. The results will run the gamut from nonsense to common sense; use your judgment and a physician's advice to figure out which is which.

The simple search word "migraine" or "headache" will net you several thousand hits during an online search, so narrow the results down by getting more specific. Here are some examples:

migraine + sumatriptan + side effects
headache + cluster + treatment
migraine + herbs + folk medicine

Be aware that not all online services use the same address. If your service provides access to the Internet, try the addresses listed here for the various organizations and websites. If you're unable to make a connection, use a search engine to find the site. And remember, no matter what its source, *online information can't replace the role of a doctor who has had the chance to get your detailed history, observed the effects of your migraine in person, and who can follow up with you on a regular basis.*

Books and Videos

Conquer Your Headaches. Robert G. Ford, M.D. and Kay T. Ford, R.N. International Headache Management, 1994.

Coping with Your Headaches. Seymour Diamond, M.D. and Mary Franklin Epstein. International Universities Press, 1982.

Headache Free. Roger Cady, M.D. and Kathleen Farmer, Psy.D. Bantam Books, 1996.

Headache Help. Lawrence Robbins, M.D. and Susan S. Lang. Houghton Mifflin, 1995.

Headacne Relief. Alan M. Rapoport, M.D. and Fred D. Sheftell, M.D. Simon & Schuster, 1991.

The Hormone Headache. Seymour Diamond, M.D., with Bill and Cynthia Still. Macmillan, 1995.

Migraine. Time-Life Home Video Series. One in a series of videos targeting specific disorders. Introduced by former Surgeon General C. Everett Koop.

Migraine: Beating the Odds. Richard B. Lipton, M.D. Lawrence C. Newman, M.D., and Helene MacLean. Addison-Wesley, 1992.

Migraine: What Works! Joseph Kandel, M.D. and David B. Sudderth, M.D. Prima Publishing, 1996.

Migraine, The Complete Guide: A Comprehensive Resource Book for People with Migraine, Their Families and Physicians. American Council for Headache Education, with Lynne M. Constantine and Suzanne Scott. Dell, 1994.

Migraine: Winning the Fight of Your Life. Charles Theisler. Starburst Publishers, 1995.

No More "Not Tonight Dear" . . . An audiocassette companion to the book *Conquer Your Headaches*, by Robert G. Ford, M.D. and Kay T. Ford, R.N. International Headache Management; 1-800-307-7246.

Taking Control of Your Headache. Paul N. Duckro, Ph.D., William D. Richardson, M.D., and Janet E. Marshall, R.N., with Steven Cassabaum and Greg Marshall. Foreword by Seymour Diamond, M.D. Guilford Press, 1995.

Index

AASH; *see* American Association for the Study of Headache (AASH)

Abdominal migraine, 26, 92
childhood migraine, form of, 98

Abortive drugs, 101–102, 132, 136, 138, 139, 143, 145, 146, 148, 152

Acetaminophen, 12, 87, 100, 135, 136
childhood migraine and, 100–101

ACHE; *see* American Council for Headache Education (ACHE)

Acupuncture, 107, 156, 157, 165–66

Adalat, 149

Advil, 78, 79, 101, 144

Alcohol, 58, 60, 63, 73, 85, 136, 137, 138, 139, 144, 149, 150, 154, 192
insomnia and, 192
trigger, as a, 192

Aleve, 101, 148

Allergies, 54, 61–62, 71, 119
Decadron Tablets used for, 140

Allopathy, 162

Alternative therapies
acupuncture; *see* Acupuncture
aromatherapy, 156, 163
autogenic training, 172
biofeedback; *see* Biofeedback
children and, 161
chiropractic, 165
diving chambers, 176
herbal remedies; *see* Herbal remedies
holistic medicine, 162–63
homeopathic remedies, 162
hypnosis, 173
meditation, 170
migraine-fighting magnets, 173–74
physical therapy, 166–67
pure oxygen, 173
relaxation techniques; *see* Relaxation techniques
seasickness wristbands, 175
TENS, 175
trigger point injections (TPT), 173–74

Ambien, 102

American Association for the Study of Headache (AASH), 117, 235

American Council for Headache Education (ACHE), 235–37

Americans with Disabilities Act, 190

Anaprox, 101, 148

241

Aneurysm, 9, 17, 51, 77, 122
Anorexia, 25, 176
Antidepressants, 132, 152
  tricyclic, 132
Antihistamines, 54, 62, 102
Aromatherapy, 156, 160
  incense, 163
Arthritis
  Decadron Tablets used for, 140
  drugs used for, 144
Aspartame, 67, 68
Aspirin, 12, 135, 149, 157, 160
  children and, 100
Asthma, 54
  beta-blockers and, 148
  Blocadren and, 153
  Decadron Tablets used for, 140
Atavan, 141
Aura, 3, 12, 26, 56, 70, 78, 111,
    151, 155
  blood flow and, 42
  causes of, 42
  children and, 94, 97–99
  classic, 13
  defined, 5
  examples of, 28–29
  food cravings and, 25
  fortification spectra, 5
  Hildegard of Bingen, 18
  hyperventilation and, 176
  macropsia, 5
  medication and, 30
  micropsia, 5
  negative scotoma, 5
  olfactory, 32
  photopsia, 5
  prevention of, 31
  prodrome, 19
  sensory, 5
  spiritual interpretations, 18
  teichopsia, 5
Autogenic training, 172
Autonomic nervous system, 43
Autosomal dominant disorder, 47
Aventyl, 102
Axotal, 138

Bayer, 137
Belladonna, 163
Bellergal, 142
Bellergal-S, 163
Benign orgasmic cephalgia, 74
Beta-blockers, 46, 75, 81, 87, 102,
    126, 132, 138, 148, 149, 151,
    153
  children and, 94, 99, 107, 108
  defined, 168
Biofeedback, 37, 59, 63, 84, 88,
    92, 93, 112, 156, 157, 158,
    168–70, 172–73, 178
  children and, 94, 99, 107, 108
  defined, 168
Birth control pills, 17, 71, 78, 80,
    85, 112
  menstrual migraine and, 86
Black poplar, 160
Blocadren, 102, 153
Blood clots, 51, 53
Blood vessels, 37, 38, 39, 44, 46,
    54, 58
  dilation of, 40, 69
  prostaglandin, effect of, 81
Brain, 44, 46, 51, 62, 73
  neurological disturbances, 41
  parts of, 38–39
  scans, 41
  stem, 39, 75
Brain tumor, 9, 11, 51, 95, 96, 122
Breast-feeding, 80
  drugs and, 150
  medications and, 88, 139
Bright-light therapy, 12
British Migraine Association, The,
    237
Butalbital, 101, 138–139

Cafatine-PB, 142
Cafergot, 83, 101, 142, 143
Caffeine, 60, 65, 66, 85, 101
  analgesics with, 132
  childhood trigger, 103
Calan, 154
Calcium channel blockers, 112,
    132, 143, 149, 153, 154
Capillaries, 41, 44
  barriers, 42

Catapres, 11, 139
CAT scan, 7, 97, 121
Cerebellum, 38
Cerebral cortex, 38
Cerebrum, 38
Cervical spine, 39
Chamomile, 160
Chemoreceptor, 43
Childhood migraine
  abdominal migraine and, 98
  abortive drugs, 101–102
  acetaminophen, 100–101
  alternative therapies, 99–100
  candy-coated medications, 102
  computer monitors, 104
  depression and, 110
  diagnosing, 95–97
  headache anger, controlling, 106
  lunch meats and, 105
  medications for, 100–102
  nausea, combating, 104
  preventive medications, 102
  rebound headache, 106
  Reye's syndrome and, 100
  school and, 108–109
  stress and, 109–10
  support groups for, 107, 110
  symptoms, recognition of, 96–98
  tetracycline, dangers of, 108
  treatment for, 93–95
  triggers, 94, 100, 103–104
  Vitamin A, dangers of, 108
Children, 8, 47
  abdominal migraine and, 26
  alternative therapies and, 161
  aura; *see* Aura
  biofeedback; *see* Biofeedback
  Blocadren and, 153
  diarrhea and, 26
  headaches, 93
  herbal remedies and, 161
  Midrin and, 136
  migraine variants, 13
  mood swings and, 98, 108
  Tigan and, 154
  triggers, 94
Chiropractic adjustments, 107, 165

Chocolate, 65, 66, 69, 85, 187
  childhood trigger, 103
Circadian rhythm, 72, 76
Circulatory system, 39
Cluster headaches, 3, 7, 10, 13, 22,
    23, 53, 133, 147
  antihistamines and, 62
  Catapres used for, 140
  causes of, 43
  children and, 98
  Depakote used for, 141
  DHE-45 used for, 141
  diving chambers and, 176
  drooping eyelids and, 24
  drugs used for, 142, 146, 150,
    153, 154
  men and, 11, 16
  pure oxygen and, 173
  sleep apnea and, 44
  steroids used for, 152
  sunlight and, 72
  treatments for, 11–12
Codeine, 87, 132
  Tylenol, with, 136
Coffee, 12, 58
Compazine, 151
Complicated migraine, 10
Computer monitors, 71, 73, 104,
    176, 189
Concomitant disorder, 50
Corgard, 148
Coronary heart disease, 90
CT scan, 121
Cyproheptadine, 83

Damiana, 161
Decadron, 83
Decadron-LA, 140
Decadron Tablets, 140
Dehydration, 26, 71, 73
  childhood trigger, 103
  trigger, as a, 65, 77, 167
Delalone D.P., 140
Deltasone, 150
Demerol, 87, 146
Depakote, 11, 141
Depression, 57, 62, 71, 102, 139

Depression *(continued)*
  children and, 110
  drugs used for, 144, 145
  Endep used for, 137
  side effect, as a, 140, 144, 145, 150
  spreading, 58
DHE, 142, 153
DHE-45, 11, 83, 141, 143, 155
Diamox, 83
Diarrhea, 26, 69
  children and, 98
  side effect, as a, 144, 145, 147, 152
Diet, 8, 68, 192
  elimination; *see* Elimination diet
  food triggers, 186
  trigger-free, 180
  vegetarian, 64
Dilantin, 102, 141
Diving chambers, 176
Dizziness, 10, 26, 28, 50, 116
  children and, 98
  side effect, as a, 136–39, 144, 145, 150, 153, 154
DNA, 50
Doctors
  choosing a, 116–17
  common questions asked by, 118–19
  common questions to ask, 119–20
  diagnostic tests, 120–23
  dissatisfaction with, 124–25
  male vs. female, 124
  types of, 115–16
  when to visit one, 114–15
Dolopine, 147
Dreaming, 75–76
Drugs
  first-line defense, 135
  list of, 135–54
  preventive; *see* Preventive drugs
  second-line defense, 135
  third-line medications, 135
Dura mater, 38

Ecotrin, 137
Edema, 25, 65
EEG; *see* Electroencephalogram (EEG)
Elavil, 102, 136
Electroencephalogram (EEG), 121
Elimination diet, 60, 103
Endep, 137
Endorphins, 45, 187
Ergomar, 83, 142
Ergonovine, 83
Ergostat, 142
Ergotamine, 75, 101, 112, 132
  breast-feeding and, 88
  tartrate, 83
Ergots, 11, 141, 148, 151, 153
ERT; *see* Estrogen replacement therapy (ERT)
Esgic, 102, 138
Eskalith, 146
Estradiol gel, 83
Estrogen, 49, 80, 81, 85, 86, 89
  patch, 83, 89, 90
  pills, 71
Estrogen replacement therapy (ERT), 89–90
Excedrin, 101, 137, 155
Exercise, 77, 84, 94, 156, 167, 180, 186–87
  children and, 110
  trigger, as a, 167
Exertion headache, 74, 77
Eye problems, 24, 54

Family coping strategies, 181–85
FAQ's (Frequently Asked Questions), 238
FDA, 49, 70, 133
Feverfew, 156, 158, 162
Fioricet, 101, 138
Fiorinal, 101, 138
  Codeine, with, 138
5-HT1, 152
Folk remedies; *see* Alternative therapies

Food
  colorings, 70
  cravings, 25
Food and Drug Administration
    (FDA); *see* FDA
Fortification spectra, 5

Garlic pills, 163
Genetics, 50, 95
Glaucoma, 51, 115, 136, 150

Hallucinations, 5, 29
  children and, 99
  side effect, as a, 147, 152
Headache anger, 106
Headache calendar, 128
Headache diary, 2, 57, 59, 66, 81,
    103, 168, 181, 183
  information included in, 128
Headache hangover, 14
Headaches, 50
  with aura, 3
  children and, 93
  chronic daily, 13
  classic, 3
  cluster; *see* Cluster headaches
  common, 3
  cyclic, 148
  exertion, 74
  hatband, 77
  hunger, 68
  hypertension, 52
  letdown, 72
  menstrual cycles and, 14
  pain, types of, 22
  post-traumatic, 53
  rating, 13, 128
  rebound; *see* Rebound headaches
  sinus, 32, 53–54
  symptom of migraine, as a, 6
  tension-type; *see* Tension-type
      headaches
  types of, 7
  unilateral; *see* Unilateral
      headaches
  without aura, 3
Head trauma, 71
Health maintenance organization
    (HMO); *see* HMO

Hemiplegic migraine, 50, 143, 153
Hepatitis, 96, 141
Herbal remedies, 156, 157–62
  children and, 161
Heredity, 47, 48
High blood pressure, 52, 64
  Catapres used for, 140
  children and, 96
Hildegard of Bingen, 18
HMO, 123–24
  treatment coverage, 129
Holistic medicine, 162–63
Homeopathic remedies, 162
Homeostasis, 49, 58, 74
Hormone replacement therapy, 90
Hormones, 49, 80, 86
HPP; *see* Hydrolyzed plant protein
    (HPP)
Hunger headaches, 68
HVP; *see* Hydrolyzed vegetable
    protein (HVP)
Hydrolyzed plant protein (HPP), 67
Hydrolyzed vegetable protein
    (HVP), 67
Hypersomnia, 75
Hypertension, 9, 52, 74, 113, 136,
    140, 153
  Tenormin used for, 138
Hypnosis, 59, 157, 173
Hypoglycemia, 52
Hypothalamus, 39, 49, 55, 68
Hysterectomy, 89, 90

Ibuprofen, 12, 101, 137, 144
Imitrex, 12, 30, 57, 79, 82, 132,
    133, 147, 152–53, 176, 178
  breast-feeding and, 88
Inderal, 75, 102, 151
Inderal-LA, 151
Indocin, 145
Indomethacin, 74, 75, 167
Insomnia, 75
  alcohol and, 192
  Endep used for, 137
  meditation and, 170
  menopause, symptom of, 89

Insomnia *(continued)*
    side effect, as a, 140, 145, 147,
        151
Insulin, 52
Insurance, 129
International Headache Society, 3,
    7
Internet, 107, 178, 184
    resources on, 237–39
    search engines, 239
Intracranial, 38
Ischemia, 42
Isoptin, 154

*Journal of American Medical
    Association (JAMA)* study, 7,
    8, 16

Ketorolac tromethamine, 83

Lemon balm, 160, 162
Lifestyle changes, 191–93
Light, 82
    changes in, 73
    flashing, 94
    patterns, changes in, 65
    sensitivity, 2, 4, 6, 14, 32, 34,
        98, 144, 146
Lithane, 146
Lithium, 11, 146
Lopressor, 148
Lumbar puncture, 122

Magnesium, 68–69
Magnetic resonance arteriography
    (MRA); *see* MRA
Magnetic resonance imaging (MRI);
    see MRI
Magnetic resonance spectography,
    121
Magnets, migraine-fighting, 174–75
MAOs; *see* Monoamine oxidase
    inhibitors (MAOs)
Marplan, 145
Massage, 21, 156, 164
Meadowsweet, 160, 162
Medihaler Ergotamine, 142
Medipren, 144

Meditation, 170
Melatonin, 49, 76, 77
Men
    cluster headaches and, 11, 16
    migraine and, 48
Menarche, 84
Meninges, 38, 46
Meningitis, 51, 95, 96, 116
Menopause, 49, 71, 80, 90
    symptoms of, 88–89
Menstrual migraine, 79, 82, 90
    birth control pills and, 86
    drugs used for, 144, 148
    non drug therapies, 84
    treatments for, 82–84
    triggers associated with, 85
Menstruation, 10, 14, 58, 71, 86
    chamomile and, 160
    trigger, as a, 81, 85
Methadone, 139
Methergine, 83
Methysergide, 132
Micropsia, 5
Midrin, 101, 136
Migraine
    abdominal; *see* Abdominal
        migraine
    age and, 54
    allergies and, 61–62
    aspartame and, 67
    aura, with, 3, 7, 30, 43
    aura, without, 3, 7, 30, 43
    basilar, 153
    basilar artery, 10–11
    blood vessels and, 38
    childhood, 47
    children and, 8, 13
    classification chart, 194–95
    complicated, 7, 10
    concomitant disorder, as a, 50
    dangers of, 9
    defined, 4
    dreaming and, 75–76
    drugs, list of, 135–54
    exertion, 77
    familial hemiplegic, 7, 50
    frequency, 13

hemiplegic, 50, 143, 153
high blood pressure and, 52
hormones, role of, 49
hypoglycemia and, 52
hypothalamus, role of, 39
identifying, 10
inherited disorder, as a, 47
intelligence and, 8
letdown, 54
medications for, list of, 135–54
men and, 48
menarche, 84
menstrual; *see* Menstrual
  migraine
menstrual cycles and, 49
multiple-organ disorder, as a, 47
myths, 112
neurovascular disorder, as a, 40
nighttime, 76
ocular symptoms, 24
onset of, 8
orgasmic, 145
pattern, 53
personality, 48
primary disorder, as a, 39, 50
prostaglandin, effect of, 81
race and, 14–15
ratings, 183
receptors and, 46
"red," 24
risks for, 55
secondary disorder, as a, 50
seratonin and, 45
sinus headache differentiated
  from, 53
socioeconomic factors, 8
stages of, 19–20
symptoms of, 6
testing for, 7
variant, 12–13
"white," 24
workplace, in the, 187–90
Migraine Foundation, The, 237
Migraine related stroke
  birth control pills and, 86
  smoking and, 87
Moduretic, 83

Monoamine oxidase inhibitors
  (MAOs), 136, 144, 145, 147,
  150, 152, 154
Monosodium glutamate (MSG);
  see MSG
Mood swings, 34
  children and, 98, 108
  side effect, as a, 142, 147, 151
Motrin, 101, 144
MRA, 121
MRI, 97, 121
MSG, 57, 59, 67, 187
  childhood trigger, 103

Nalfon, 143
Naprosyn, 101, 149
Naproxen, 149
Nardil, 147, 150
National Headache Foundation
  (NHF), 117, 232–35
  support groups, network of, 234
Nausea, 4, 6, 10, 12–13, 14, 26,
  32, 42, 50, 56, 69, 78, 82,
  111, 115, 132, 145
  cerebellum, role of, 39
  children and, 104
  drugs used for, 146, 148, 151
  Imitrex used for, 79
  seasickness wristbands and, 175
  side effect, as a, 138, 139, 142,
  147, 152, 154
  Thorazine used for, 139
Negative scotoma, 5
Neuroimaging, 7, 121
Neurontin, 143
Neurotransmitter, 45
Newsgroups, 238
NHF; *see* National Headache
  Foundation (NHF)
Nimotop, 149
Nitrates, 70
Nitrites, 70
Nitroglycerin, 31, 74
Noise, 71, 72
Nonsteroidal anti-inflammatory
  drugs (NSAIDs); *see* NSAIDs
Noradrenaline, 45

NSAIDs, 93, 131, 143–46, 149, 153
list of, 83
Numbness, 2
face and limbs, 10
hands and feet, 5, 14, 98, 149
side effect, as a, 142, 144
Nuprin, 101, 144

Odors, 70
Opioids, 132, 154
Orudis, 145
Osteoporosis, 89
side effect, as a, 152
Over-the-counter (OTC) drugs, 101, 113, 114, 128, 131, 148, 155
analgesics, 132
Oxygen, 73
pure, 12, 173

Pamelor, 102, 150
Paralysis, temporary, 2, 10, 50
Passionflower, 160–61
Peptides, 66, 69
Periactin, 83, 102, 140
Pesticides, 71
PET scan, 122
Phenergan, 83, 104
Phenobarbital, 102
Phonophobia, 32
Photophobia, 32
Photopsia, 5
Phrenilin, 101, 138
Phrenilin Forte, 138
Physical therapy, 166
Physician's Desk Reference, 133
Pia mater, 38, 46
Pill Book, The, 133
Placebo, 140, 159
response, 157
PMS; *see* Premenstrual syndrome (PMS)
Porphyria, 139, 140
Positron emission tomography (PET); *see* PET scan

Postdrome, 20, 21, 32
Prednisone, 141
Pregnancy, 49, 80, 88
migraines and, 87–88
passionflower and, 161
Premenstrual syndrome (PMS), 79, 82, 85, 112
Preventive drugs
types of, 132–33
Primary disorder, 39, 50
Primrose oil, 161
Procardia, 149
Procardia XL, 149
Prodrome, 19, 20, 33
food cravings and, 25
Progesterone, 49, 80, 85, 89, 90
Propanolol, 83
Prophylactics, 132, 150, 151
Prostaglandins, 62, 80, 138, 145, 148, 153
Prozac, 144, 152
Puberty, 80, 84, 93

Radio-frequency trigeminal gangliolysis, 12
Rebound headaches, 10, 13, 21, 66, 145
children and, 94, 106
defined, 14
side effect, as a, 136, 137, 139, 141, 144, 147, 150, 153
Red-dye #40, 69–70
childhood trigger, 103
Red migraine, 24
Red wine, 58, 59, 63, 70
Referred pain, 42–43, 53
Reglan, 83, 148
Relaxation techniques, 49, 63, 72, 88, 119, 157, 169, 170–72, 180, 192
children and, 94, 100, 108
workplace, in the, 188
Rescue drugs, 132, 148
Reye's syndrome, 100, 137
Ronda's Home Page, 238
Rufen, 144

Sandomigran, 150
Sansert, 147
Sansert, 83
Scans
  Cat scan, 121
  CT scan, 121
  Magnetic resonance
      arteriography (MRA), 121
  PET scan, 122
Scotoma, 126
Secondary disorder, 50
Sensory aura, 5
Seratonin, 76, 147, 152, 158
  defined, 45
  receptors, 69
  regulation of, 142
Sibelium, 143
Sinus headaches, 53–54
Sinusitis, 95
Sleep, 55
  apnea, 44, 75, 76
  hypothalamus, role of, 39, 49
  patterns, 71
  stages, 76
Smoking, 60, 73, 87, 191
Sodium, 59, 64
Sodium nitrite, 70
Sound sensitivity, 4, 6, 34
Sparine, 151
Speech, slurred, 30, 51, 116
  children and, 98
Spinal cord, 39, 51, 75
Spinal tap, 122
Spreading depression, 58
Stadol, 139
Steroids, 49, 152
Stomach upset, 92, 101
  drugs used for, 144, 148, 154
  side effect, as a, 142, 148, 152
Stress, 54, 57, 61, 62, 71
  children, trigger in, 94, 103, 109–
      10
Stroke, 42, 51
  migraine related, 86
Subdermal hematoma, 51, 53
Sulfites, 63, 70, 136
Sumatriptan; *see* Imitrex
Sunlight, 71, 72

Support groups, 16, 35, 107, 178,
      179, 181, 184, 232
  children and, 110
  National Headache Foundation
      (NHF) network of, 234
Symptoms, 4, 6
  invisible, 3

Tannins, 162
Teichopsia, 5
Temporal arteritis, 54
Temporomandibular joint
      syndrome (TMJ), 23, 53, 95,
      121
Tenormin, 138
TENS, 175
Tension-type headaches, 3, 7, 13,
      17, 23, 43, 133
  children and, 98
  massage and, 21
  medications used for, 135, 136,
      138
  primrose oil and, 161
  symptoms of, 12
Tetracycline, 108
Theobromides, 66
Thermography, 122
Thorazine, 139
Tigan, 104, 153
TMJ; *see* Temporomandibular joint
      syndrome (TMJ)
Toradol, 146
Transcendental meditation (TM), 170
Transcutaneous electrical nerve
      stimulation (TENS); *see*
      TENS
Travel, 57, 58, 71, 72
  airline, 73–74
  childhood trigger, 103
Tricyclic antidepressants, 132
Trigger point injections (TPT), 173–
      74
Triggers, 34, 128
  activities acting as, 203
  alcohol, 192
  allergies, 54, 61–62
  anxiety, 49
  birth control pills, 86

Triggers (*continued*)
blood vessels, changes in, 58
bread, 64
caffeine, 65, 103
children; *see* Childhood migraine
chocolate, 66, 103
citrus fruits, 64
common, chart of, 197–202
dehydration, 65, 77, 103, 167
drugs, 74
elimination of, 59, 193
environmental, 203
estrogen, drop in, 88
excitement, 103
exercise, 167
fluorescent lights, 189
food, 2, 58, 84, 85
food colorings, 70
fragrances, 70
head trauma, 70
hormonal, 203–204
hormone replacements, 90
hunger, 186
identification of, 57, 59–61
list of, 71
low blood sugar, 52
magnesium, 69
menstruation, 81, 85
MSG, 67, 103
nitrates, 70
nitrites, 70
odors, 32, 70
overeating, 186
pollution, 71
ponytail, 77, 103
psychological, 203
puberty, 84
red dye #40, 69–70, 103
red wine, 70
role of, 48
scents, 163, 189
smoking, 73
sodium, 65
stress, 8, 10, 62–63, 85, 123, 156
sulfites, 70
travel, 71, 103
yeast extract, 64
yellow dye #5, 70, 103

Tylenol, 101, 135
Codeine, with, 136
Tyramine, 15, 62, 63, 145

Ultram, 154
Unilateral headaches, 4, 23
nausea and vomiting, 82

Valerian, 161
Valium, 140–41
Vascular system, 39, 41, 47
Vasoconstrictor, 153
Imitrex as a, 152
Vasodilators, 31
Verapomil, 79
Verelan, 154
Vervain, 161, 162
Visualization, 172
Vitamin A, 108, 174
Vitamin D, 174
Vomiting, 2, 4, 6, 10, 12–13, 14,
26, 32, 42, 50, 82, 92, 96,
100, 115, 132, 145, 155
cerebellum, role of, 39
children and, 98
drugs used for, 148, 151, 154
Imitrex used for, 79
self-induced, 176
side effect, as a, 142, 147, 154
Thorazine used for, 139

Water pills, 83
White migraine, 24
Wigraine, 83, 142
Wolff-Parkinson White syndrome,
154

Xylocaine, 11, 146

Yeast, 64
Yellow dye #5, 70
childhood trigger, 103
Yoga, 171

Zoloft, 152